Becoming a Reflective Practitioner

A reflective and holistic approach to clinical nursing, practice development and clinical supervision

Christopher Johns

with postscript from **Jean Watson**

**Blackwell
Science**

© 2000 by
Blackwell Science Ltd
Editorial Offices:
Osney Mead, Oxford OX2 0EL
25 John Street, London WC1N 2BS
23 Ainslie Place, Edinburgh EH3 6AJ
350 Main Street, Malden
  MA 02148 5018, USA
54 University Street, Carlton
  Victoria 3053, Australia
10, rue Casimir Delavigne
  75006 Paris, France

Other Editorial Offices:
Blackwell Wissenschafts-Verlag GmbH
Kurfürstendamm 57
10707 Berlin, Germany

Blackwell Science KK
MG Kodenmacho Building
7–10 Kodenmacho Nihombashi
Chuo-ku, Tokyo 104, Japan

Iowa State University Press
A Blackwell Science Company
2121 S. State Avenue
Ames, Iowa 50014-8300, USA

The right of the Author to be
identified as the Author of this Work
has been asserted in accordance
with the Copyright, Designs and
Patents Act 1988.

First published 2000
Reprinted 2001

Set in 10/12.5 pt Sabon
by DP Photosetting, Aylesbury, Bucks
Printed and bound in Great Britain by
The Alden Group, Oxford and
Northampton

The Blackwell Science logo is
a trade mark of Blackwell Science Ltd,
registered at the United Kingdom
Trade Marks Registry

DISTRIBUTORS

Marston Book Services Ltd
PO Box 269
Abingdon
Oxon OX14 4YN
(*Orders*: Tel: 01235 465500
          Fax: 01235 465555)

USA
Blackwell Science, Inc.
Commerce Place
350 Main Street
Malden, MA 02148 5018
(*Orders*: Tel: 800 759 6102
                781 388 8250
         Fax: 781 388 8255)

Canada
Login Brothers Book Company
324 Saulteaux Crescent
Winnipeg, Manitoba R3J 3T2
(*Orders*: Tel: 204 837 2987)

Australia
Blackwell Science Pty Ltd
54 University Street
Carlton, Victoria 3053
(*Orders*: Tel: 03 9347 0300
          Fax: 03 9347 5001)

A catalogue record for this title
is available from the British Library

ISBN 0-632-05561-8

Library of Congress
Cataloging-in-Publication Data
Johns, Christopher.
    Becoming a reflective practitioner : a
reflective and holistic approach to clinical
nursing, practice development, and clinical
supervision/Christopher Johns ; with a
postscript from Jean Watson.
        p. ; cm.
    Includes bibliographical references and
index.
    ISBN 0-632-05561-8 (pbk.)
    1. Nursing–Philosophy.   2. Holistic
nursing.   I. Title.
    [DNLM: 1. Philosophy, Nursing.
2. Holistic Nursing.   3. Models, Nursing.
WY 86 J65b 2000]
    RT84.5 .J636 2000
    610.73′01–dc21
                                    99-046382

For further information on
Blackwell Science, visit our website:
www.blackwell-science.com

Becoming a Reflective Practitioner

Other books of interest

Reflective Practice in Nursing
The Growth of the Professional Practitioner
Second Edition
Edited by Sarah Burns and Chris Bulman
0-632-05291-0

Mentoring, Preceptorship and Clinical Supervision
A Guide to Professional Roles in Clinical Practice
Second Edition
Alison Morton-Cooper and Anne Palmer
0-632-04967-7

Successful Supervision in Health Care Practice
Promoting Professional Development
Edited by Jenny Spouse and Liz Redfern
0-632-05159-9

Contents

Introduction

The notion of nursing, health visiting and midwifery is challenged periodically by ideas that promise much regarding the development of clinical practice. Models of nursing exemplify this trend. Yet in terms of your own experience, consider whether models of nursing have made a difference to clinical practice. As an ideal construct, a model of nursing would seem to offer much yet, when accommodated into the practice culture, it is more likely to be distorted to fit the status quo than to challenge it. Luker (1988) noted:

> 'The advantage of models based on activities of living is that they are easy to understand and fit in with the personal value systems of many nurses.' (p. 28)

As a consequence the impact is minimal; worse, it is disruptive.

A more recent innovation is reflective practice. Yet what will we make of reflective practice? Will it merely scratch the surface of practitioners' thoughts and consequently make no significant impact on developing practice? If so, the scratch will feel like an irritant and reflective practice will be rejected. In a world dominated by a technological approach to education and health care, reflective practice is at risk of being perceived and understood as merely another educational technology. Whilst it is true that reflective practice offers a valuable cognitive problem-solving model, such a limited perception fails to grasp the essential nature of reflective practice as a holistic process of learning, grounded in the whole being of the practitioner within the particular context of lived experience.

The following questions are central to this book: What does it mean to be a reflective practitioner? How does a reflective practitioner view and respond within clinical practice? What sort of structures are significant to nurture and sustain the growth of the reflective practitioner? How can reflection help practitioners to realise desirable practice, given that most practitioners strive to be holistic?

In response to these challenging questions, the Burford NDU model (Johns, 1994) is used as an exemplar of a reflective and holistic model for nursing. Reflective practice *is* holistic practice because:

- it focuses primarily on the whole experience and then seeks to understand the significance within the whole;

- it is grounded in the meaning the individual practitioner gives to that experience and seeks to facilitate such understanding;
- it acknowledges that the practitioner is ultimately self-determining and responsible for his or her destiny and seeks to facilitate this growth;
- it parallels the therapeutic intent within clinical practice and guided reflection.

It is important to emphasise that the Burford NDU model is simply a template for the development of an appropriate reflective model. Unlike more traditional models of nursing, it does not intend to prescribe or impose a reality of nursing. The reflective reader will be informed and guided by this exemplar in constructing their own reflective model. To construct a reflective model, practitioners need to:

- reflect on the validity of their existing philosophy for practice;
- revise their philosophy to provide a clear, detailed, dynamic vision for practice that reflects shared understandings;
- adapt the Burford NDU cues in constructing an adequate series of reflective cues to tune into their own beliefs and values within each unfolding clinical moment;
- adapt the underlying philosophical assumptions.

Alternatively, the Burford model can be utilised as presented in this book.

I have tried to write the book in a reflective style through the stories written in my reflective journal and those which practitioners have shared with me in guided reflection. As a consequence, I have not always drawn out the significance of issues within the practitioners' reflective accounts and dialogue. Where I have provided interpretations, then these are only my view. Readers may draw out other interpretations based on their own experiences. Indeed, I encourage the reader to ask 'what does this mean to me?' and 'how do I relate to this in terms of my own experience?'. Rather than see the text as prescriptive I encourage readers to view the text as a source of information to help them reflect on their own practice, given that stories are always subjective and contextual. You, the reader, will find your own meanings and reflect on and make sense of them in the context of your own experience. This approach may feel very different from that of conventional text books where theory is set out in a more orderly way.

The reflective practitioner has an open and curious mind, free from constraining attitudes and prejudices, in order to see or read the thing for what it is. I have endeavoured to draw the reader's attention to significant issues and prompt reflection through challenging questions. Given the prevailing widespread use of prescriptive and reductive models of nursing and the infancy of reflective thought for many practitioners, it is easy to view the Burford model through a prescriptive lens. To prescribe how practitioners should believe and act would be a contradiction within a reflective paradigm. As a consequence, the reader is challenged to read the book with what Dewey (1933) refers to as a sceptical eye:

> 'Reflective action entails active and persistent consideration of any belief or supposed form of knowledge in the light of the grounds that support it and the consequences to which it leads.' (p. 215)

As with all sources of theory, its purpose is to inform the reader's own personal theories. Nurses, with their responsibility to be most effective, are obliged to consider the value of extant theory within the context of their own practice. From a reflective perspective, theory only has value in context. I have endeavoured to portray theory through practitioners' reflective accounts or stories of everyday practice. Stories are, by their very nature, subjective and contextual, connected to previous stories within an unbroken flow of experience over time. The stories are also emotional, reflecting the intimacy, anguish and joy of human encounter. The stories are complex and contradictory, reflecting the complex, indeterminate nature of much of clinical practice. As such, the stories do not necessarily have a logical flow, rational argument, neat endings or, indeed, any endings at all but often raise more questions as threads that extend the stories into an unpredictable future.

The development of this approach has been established through a collaborative and ongoing research process that commenced in 1989 (Johns, 1998a). The beauty of story is the way it illuminates the contextual meaning of complex theory in ways that the reader can sense and feel in the context of their own experience. Story telling:

- illuminates the subtlety and complexity of caring and theory as a whole. This is significant from a holistic perspective;
- makes visible the nuances and significance of caring within the mundaneness of everyday practice;
- 'tests' the meaningfulness of extant theory within the unfolding caring situation;
- invites the listener or reader to relate to the story in terms of their own experience.

Structure of the book

The Burford model, like most models of nursing, is underpinned by a number of explicit philosophical assumptions about the nature of nursing (Box 1). These assumptions are abstract statements that have been retrospectively constructed. By 'retrospective' I mean that a reflective model begins with

Box 1   The Burford NDU model: explicit assumptions of caring in practice (Johns, 1998a).

- Caring in practice is grounded in a valid philosophy for practice underpinned by the unifying concept of human caring (Roach, 1992; Watson, 1988).
- All persons are seen and responded to as unitary human beings (Rogers, 1986).
- The intent of nursing is to enable the other to realise recovery and growth as expanding consciousness (Newman, 1994), through appropriate caring–healing responses.
- The nurse works with the other through a continuing advocacy dialogue (Gadow, 1980) mirrored by an internal dialogue with self (reflection-within-the-moment).
- Caring in practice is made manifest, known and developed through reflection-on-experience.
- Realisation of caring in practice is determined by the extent to which the practitioner is available to work with the other (Johns, 1996a).
- Growth is a mutual process of realisation.
- Caring in practice is a responsive and reflexive form in the context of the environment in which it is practised.

---

reflection on lived experience and, through a process of analysis, the underlying theory is made explicit and is informed by extant theory as appropriate. This is a natural process of dynamic evolution whereby the emergent theory is constantly reflected on for its appropriateness. Philosophical assumptions are significant in the context of theory development; they are the necessary interlocking parts of a complex, holistic view of nursing. Each part is significant in its own right, yet cannot be viewed in isolation from the whole. This is the essential notion of holism that challenges a reductionist approach towards nursing and health care, which contends that parts of the whole can be seen in isolation.

These explicit assumptions provide the structure for the book. Chapter 1 sets out the essential nature of a philosophy or vision for practice and its core significance within a template for a reflective model for nursing. The nature of holistic caring theory implied in the explicit assumptions is explored, and the influence of nursing philosophers – Simone Roach, Jean Watson, Martha Rogers, Margaret Newman and Lydia Hall – is considered. By drawing on their work, the significance of nursing theory is acknowledged in the way it informs practice without prescribing what nurses ought to be.

The reader may feel that some of this theory is far removed from practice, yet theory always underpins practice in some guise. As such, I urge the reader to engage theory and not to feel intimidated by this work. Remember, the book is a reference, a source of information.

Chapter 2 discusses the nature and significance of establishing an existential reflective dialogue between the practitioner and the patient and family. The intention of the dialogue is to establish the practitioner–patient relationship whereby the practitioner can be available to work with the patient and family to help them meet their health needs.

Chapter 3 outlines the essential nature of being a reflective practitioner and the process of guided reflection as a developmental process, congruent with holistic practice. A model for nursing should pay attention to the developmental process required for practitioners to become skilled in putting the model into practice. Therefore many of the stories shared within the book are constructed through dialogue in order to illustrate the process of guiding reflection. The reader is encouraged to view each dialogue from three perspectives:

(1) in terms of the self's own experience and practice;
(2) to imagine what it is like for the practitioner to share their story within guided reflection;
(3) to reflect on the process of guided reflection.

This chapter also considers the emergence of clinical supervision and the way guided reflection can structure the clinical supervision space and relationship.

Chapter 4 reveals the significance of the assumption that *the extent to which nurses (practitioners) can realise caring in practice is determined by the extent to which they are available to work with the person (to help them meet their health needs)*. The extent to which the practitioner can be available is determined by six criteria:

(1) knowing what is desirable;
(2) concern for the other;
(3) knowing the person;
(4) the aesthetic response;
(5) knowing and managing self's involvement within relationships;
(6) creating and sustaining an environment where being available is possible.

The significance of the first three criteria is explored. The significance of reflective journalling as a therapeutic tool for patients is illuminated and discussed through the story of Moira Vass, a woman who journalled her anguish of living and eventually died from motor neurone disease.

Chapter 5 explores the significance of the practitioner responding effectively within an unfolding clinical situation. The emphasis of reflection is not on technical apects of care but, rather, difficult relational issues.

Chapter 6 explores the significance of knowing and managing self's involvement within relationships. Simon Lee's reflective account illuminates and reflects on his relationship with Bill, a patient with a terminal illness, and Bill's family. Simon's story is characterised by his own suffering and his effort to put his feelings into a meaningful perspective. Holistic practitioners view themselves as a therapeutic tool in working with patients and families. To respond to the patient's and the family's emotional needs requires the nurse to engage on an emotional and intimate level that may provoke considerable anxiety. The effective practitioner learns to manage involvement without diminishing concern or intimacy.

Chapter 7 explores the significance of creating and sustaining an environment where being available is possible. This chapter gives insight into the meaning and development of holistic practice. It also deals with the conditions of practice which practitioners perceive as limiting the realisation of holistic practice as a lived reality, such as interpersonal relationships and the realities of NHS management.

Chapter 8 explores written and oral reflective communication within the premise that communication needs to be both practical and meaningful. The book is concluded by a postscript or reflection by Jean Watson, whose work has been a constant source of wisdom and inspiration along my own reflective and caring journey.

The explicit assumption, '*Caring in practice is a responsive and reflexive form in context of the environment in which it is practised*', reflects the way I have tried to write this book, by drawing on the Burford NDU model as an exemplar and template for a reflective and holistic model for nursing, although clearly, there are other ways of constructing such a model. A reflective model is always dynamic and evolves as practitioners develop practice. The model needs to create a tension between offering a vision for practice and a reflection of reality. Although the holistic and reflective model has been developed against a nursing background, it is a significant model for all health-care practitioners. For this reason I endeavour to use the word 'practitioner' in preference to 'nurse' throughout the text. Where I have used the word 'nurse' it can be exchanged for 'health-care practitioner'. The pronoun 'her' is used to represent the practitioner.

Christopher Johns

Acknowledgements

To Valerie Young for her friendship and her persistent and invaluable critical reading of draft manuscripts.
To Simon Lee and Moira Vass for their stories.
To Jean Watson for her work and for her continuous encouragement and inspiration to myself and to nursing.
To all the practitioners who worked with me within guided reflection and whose stories illuminate and give meaning to theory.
To Griselda Campbell at Blackwell Science for her support and for having faith.
To my family for their endurance.

My acknowledgment and thanks for permission to reprint versions of stories previously published:

Tom's story (p. 11) in *Nursing Inquiry* (1998) **5**, 18–24. Caring through a reflective lens: giving meaning to being a reflective practitioner.

Jade's story with Molly (p. 72) and Hilda (p. 139) in the *Journal of Clinical Nursing* (1993) **3**, 307–12. On becoming effective in taking ethical action.

Janet and Michelle's story (p. 126) in *Nursing Standard* (1996) **11**, 34–8. Using a reflective model of nursing and guided reflection.

Leslie's story with Alec in the *Journal of Advanced Nursing* (1996) **24**, 1135–43.

Mavis and Joy (p. 144) in the *Journal of Clinical Nursing* (1993) **2**, 89–93. Learning through supervision: a case study of respite care.

Remembering Moira Vass.

Chapter 1

Constructing a Philosophy for Practice

At the core of any reflective model of nursing is a vision or philosophy of practice. From a reflective perspective, the vision is a reflection of practitioners' beliefs and values about the nature of their practice. A philosophy is a collective statement of shared beliefs and values that are congruent with the practice setting that gives both meaning and direction to everyday practice: a light to show the way.

Where groups of practitioners work together it is evident that they need to share a common belief system in order to ensure a consistent approach towards patients and families. A written statement becomes a public statement to which others – patients, families, society as a whole and other health-care workers – can relate. It sets up the possibility for dialogue and collaboration. Indeed, the *process* of writing the philosophy gives nurses the opportunity to discuss collectively the meaning of their practice. This process promotes a dynamic practice environment in which beliefs are constantly challenged and clarified for their meaning and relevance. The philosophy, as a vision for practice, becomes the foundation stone for all clinical practice and practice development. Through common ownership, each individual practitioner's right to express her beliefs and values is acknowledged. Everyone holds beliefs about the world which are important to them and *should* strongly influence the way they respond to practice. I emphasise *should* because often nurses compromise their beliefs within health-care environments governed by the values of more dominant organisational and medical influences.

Challenging the functional conception of defining nursing

One difficulty nurses seem to have with writing a philosophy for practice is that their perception of what nursing is has been dominated by a functional rather than a philosophical conception.

1

Functional perspective   Philosophical perspective
Nursing defined in terms ⟷ Nursing defined in terms
of what nurses do   of practitioners' beliefs and values

Perhaps one reason why nursing has been so functional is that it has generally been organised through prescribed tasks beneath the shadow of a dominant belief culture of the medical model. This model reduces people to the status of patients with a series of symptoms, with subsequent medical diagnosis labels that indicate the treatment response. Within this culture, nurses have suspended their own beliefs as relatively unimportant. This parallels suspension of the rights of people expected to respond as good patients to investigation and treatment regimens. Nursing's primary role has been to support this endeavour. Caring has become a subculture, furtively taking place alongside the real work of supporting the medical programme. As such, nursing as caring has not been valued by the organisation and even by nurses themselves. If this is true, then writing a philosophy for practice is an opportunity for nurses to give voice to and assert their nursing/caring beliefs. It begins a process of empowerment that is central to reflective practice.

Unfortunately, the prevailing functional approach to British nursing has led to an attitude that writing a philosophy is some kind of window dressing. Perhaps this attitude has been encouraged by the English National Board for Nursing, Health Visiting and Midwifery (ENB) requisite that all practice areas should have a philosophy to gain approval as suitable learning environments. Although most nursing units comply with the idea of writing a philosophy of care, these philosophies do not seem to profoundly influence caring. These statements have often been written in vague rhetoric by the ward sister some years previously and are found pinned on office walls, often covered by layers of organisational memos. The rhetoric is usually grounded in caring clichés, reflecting a prevailing ideology of holistic practice that has no real meaning for practitioners and is clearly contradicted by actual practice.

Constructing a valid philosophy

When I challenged the staff at Burford Community Hospital to reflect on the meaning of nursing within the hospital, I first asked them to tell me about the hospital philosophy. They struggled to respond to this question. At this time the hospital philosophy was 'imported', based on Lydia Hall's philosophy as practised within the Loeb Center in New York (Hall, 1964; Alfano, 1971). Hall's work was a vision of nursing as a primary therapy in its own right, alongside a complementary and supportive role to medicine. From the nurses' responses it was apparent that this vision had faded. Practitioners could vaguely remember bits of it. I realised that the *imported* philosophy had imposed some sort of reality on practitioners which had denied the articulation of their own beliefs and values.

My response was to facilitate the construction of a philosophy for practice, a written statement to give purpose to nursing practice as both an individual and collective endeavour. The result (fourth edition) is shown in Box 1.1. It is the fourth edition because it evolved through reflection on its value to guide practice. Structures are always evolving in order to be adequate representations of desirable reality.

Box 1.1   Burford philosophy for practice (4th edition, January 1997).

> We believe that care is centred in the needs of the patient. The practitioner works with the patient as person, from a basis of concern and mutual understanding, where the person's experience and need for control in their life is acknowledged. In this way trust is developed between the person and the practitioner. The person is seen and responded to as a unitary human being, which includes all the person's social and cultural world.
>
> Effective care is the first priority of this hospital. Caring is holistic and intended to enable the person towards recovery and growth of health through rehabilitation, respite care, loss or dying.
>
> The hospital is integral with the community and responds to and promotes the community's needs, whether in the hospital or in the person's own home. Assessment is carried out with sensitivity in a non-intrusive manner grounded in understanding the meaning of the event for the person.
>
> Through the hospital's status as a clinical practice development unit, we accept a responsibility to continually strive to improve our caring. By appropriate monitoring and sharing, we contribute to the development of the societal value of other nurses and health-care workers.
>
> Our caring is enhanced when we mutually respect and care for each other within our respective roles. This means being free to share our feelings openly but appropriately, acknowledging that as persons, we are stressed and have differences of opinion at times. This is the basis of the therapeutic team that is essential to reciprocate and support our caring.
>
> (Adapted from draft 3, January 1997)

The original philosophy was constructed by inviting the practitioners to write on two sheets of 'flipchart' what they believed nursing at Burford Hospital was about. More and more statements were added to the sheets over the next three months. I then word processed the statements and gave each practitioner a copy. These statements were discussed during two staff meetings, resulting in a composite statement. This was eventually agreed and became accepted as the hospital philosophy. In constructing the fourth edition, some language was changed to acknowledge my own development. As I have not worked at Burford for six years, this has inevitably shifted the philosophy into a more abstract field, once removed from its fertile breeding ground. The Burford model has been placed within new contexts as I worked with other practitioners from diverse backgrounds, enabling them to find meaning in their experience of working with the model.

As you read the Burford philosophy, remember it is not your philosophy. It belongs to others and needs to be respected even though you may find parts of it you do not like. The philosophy must articulate in enough detail what is necessary to fulfil its function of giving meaning and direction to practice.

The four cornerstones

To ensure its credibility or validity, I have suggested that a philosophy for practice has four cornerstones (Johns, 1994) (Box 1.2). Of these cornerstones, the *nature of caring* sets out what is desirable, the way the practitioner hopes to practise. While I have suggested that the philosophy stems from the practitioners' own beliefs and values, such beliefs are influenced by a broad theoretical and philosophical literature. This influence on the Burford philosophy is set out below.

Box 1.2   Four cornerstones of a valid philosophy for practice.

- *The nature of caring*
This relates to the meaning that practitioners give practice in terms of therapeutic work processes and outcomes.

- *The significance of the practice context (previously the external environment of practice)*
This relates to the health-care context of the unit. In other words, what does the unit exist to do? This leads to a 'tailor-made' philosophy that pays attention to significant issues surrounding particular groups of people requiring health care.

- *The internal environment of practice*
This relates to the way nursing and health care are organised and the relationships that exist within the workplace that influence the ability of the practitioner to act in congruence with her caring beliefs. This cornerstone helps the practitioner to consider the real world to ensure the philosophy does not become merely some ideal fantasy that is patently unrelated to the messy everyday world of practice.

- *Social viability*
This relates to wider societal and professional issues to which practitioners need to pay attention in order to develop the significance of nursing and health care within society.

Yet is is important to emphasise that a philosophy is not an ideal statement. Whilst it sets out what is desirable, it must also be a reflection of reality, particularly if you accept that the philosophy is a public statement of intent. Practitioners do not practise in a context-free environment. Paying attention to the significance of the practice context prompts practitioners to contexualise their beliefs in terms of the health-care role of the unit.

Burford is a community hospital with a clearly defined health-care role.

The *internal environment of practice* prompts the practitioners to pay attention to those factors that prevent the achievement of desirable practice. Writing the philosophy gives practitioners the opportunity to begin a process of understanding their practice environment and what needs to be done in order for the philosophy to become a lived reality.

Social viability

Social viability was explained by Dorothy Johnson (1974) in terms of the three following criteria.

(1) Social congruence – Do nursing decisions and actions which are based on the philosophy fulfil social expectations or might society be helped to develop such expectations?
(2) Social significance – Do nursing decisions and actions based on the philosophy lead to outcomes for patients that make an important difference to their lives and well-being?
(3) Social utility – Is the conceptual system of the model sufficiently well developed to provide a clear direction for nursing practice, education and research?

These questions challenge practitioners to look beyond the immediate context of the practice setting towards the wider social and professional communities. The philosophy is a public statement that challenges society to 'see' nursing differently, as making a significant contribution to health care. This is important considering that many people may perceive nursing as simply supporting medicine, the ubiquitous 'doctor's handmaiden'.

A major reason why it is so important for nursing to consider its role within the particular context of health care is that health-care settings are usually determined by medical function which influences the conditions of caring. Burford is a community hospital which has a specialised function within society, including working with families in respite care, terminal care and rehabilitation. Hence caring is influenced by specialised knowledge that responds to particular need. What is effective respite care? What is effective terminal care? What is effective rehabilitation? Clearly, to respond appropriately to emerging need, the nurse needs to be suitably informed and take an active and leading role in determining the answers to these questions.

To reorientate society to value nursing requires positive action, yet positive action is also required to ensure that society's 'new' perception of nursing is constantly reinforced by nurses living out the philosophy through their everyday dialogue and actions. To know whether nursing responds to the needs of society and makes a difference requires programmes of development, evaluation and research that can appropriately demonstrate this. Social utility parallels social congruence and significance in terms of the value of the philosophy for nursing. It challenges nurses to pay attention to 'their' vision in contrast to the wider ideology of nursing.

Clearly, a valid philosophy needs to be accepted within the broad understanding of how nursing perceives itself. Burford's philosophy reflects a holistic ideology to which nurses generally subscribe. In its role as a nursing development unit (NDU), Burford accepted a commitment to be a leading edge in structuring and developing the emerging role of nursing; this book is a realisation of that commitment. Hopefully, its contribution to nursing knowledge will be acknowledged. The consequence of social viability is that nurses need to pay careful attention to the way they express their ideas within the philosophy in order for the concepts to be understood without ambiguity.

The nature of caring

Understanding the nature of holistic practice cannot be an arbitrary affair. The influence of holistic theory on the development of the Burford philosophy is set out in three assumptions that provide the philosophical and ontological foundation for holistic caring in practice.

(1)   Caring in practice is grounded in a valid philosophy for practice, underpinned by the unifying concept of human caring.
(2)   All persons are seen and responded to as unitary human beings.
(3)   The intent of nursing is to enable the other to realise recovery and growth as expanding consciousness through appropriate caring-healing responses.

In considering the significance of each of these assumptions I challenge the practitioner to reflect on the significance of this work in relation to her own beliefs and values. Clearly, there is a much greater volume of nursing theory that might have informed the Burford philosophy and which may influence your own practice. By omission, I do not mean to suggest that other texts are less relevant.

Caring in practice is grounded in a valid philosophy for practice underpinned by the unifying concept of human caring

To different extents, all professions profess to care so it is important to know what caring means within a nursing perspective. Whilst numerous authors have attempted to define caring, the influence of Morse *et al.* (1991), Kramer (1990), Watson (1988) and Halldórsdóttir (1996) is outlined below.

Ways in which caring can be conceived

Morse *et al.* (1991), in analysing the way theorists have depicted caring, characterised five ways that caring can be perceived (Box 1.3). However,

Box 1.3   Ways in which caring can be conceived (Morse *et al.*, 1991).

- As a human trait – something which is naturally part of the condition of being human
- As a moral imperative – as a fundamental virtue or value
- As an affect – extending oneself towards one's patients beyond one's job description
- As an interpersonal interaction – as something which exists tetween one person and another
- As a therapeutic – an intervention deliberately planned with a goal in mind

---

defining caring remains elusive simply because it is everything the practitioner does. To reduce caring to parts or processes is merely an effort to gain a conceptual grasp; that it might be known, or taught or researched so it can be explained or controlled in some way. Whilst Morse *et al.*'s analysis of caring may provide new perspectives to challenge the nurse, it creates an impression that caring is something different depending on the way the nurse perceives it.

Consider how Morse *et al.* might characterise the Burford philosophy. Clearly, fitting caring to types has no value except to satisfy Morse *et al.*'s own reductionist epistemological agenda concerned with defining caring as some abstract fixed entity so it can be practised, taught and researched with (false) certainty. Their typology merely reflects the elusiveness of defining caring. Caring can only ever be known on an ontological level within the unfolding caring moment.

Working with the person

Central to the Burford philosophy is the concept of *working with the person*. The essence of 'working with' is captured by Kramer (1990) in her account of holistic nursing.

> 'The holistic view holds the individual ultimately responsible for health, and individuals are deemed both capable and responsible for choosing experiences that will enhance health. In the holistic view, the health care provider is not in a detached power relation to the patient. Rather, both are active and committed participants in enhancing growth towards health.' (cited in Johns, 1994 p. 24)

Kramer's words help to focus the caring relationship around the meaning the person gives to health and responsibility. The concept of *committed participants* emphasises working with the other yet from a real sense of commitment that this person and their experience is of great significance. Kramer also helps to extend the vision of holism beyond the idea that the whole is greater than the sum of its parts.

The notion of the practitioner knowing the person as a whole is an important consideration. What does this mean? First and foremost, it is significant in acknowledging *the person* rather than *a patient* in the sense of countering the pervasive influence of the medical model which has traditionally reduced a person to the social and medical status of a patient in search of a diagnosis. This usually involves a search of the body systems until the cause is found in order for a treatment to be prescribed. This approach has been criticised because it separates the body from the whole person, leading to a lack of attention to the spiritual, psychological, emotional and social impact on the person and family. It is also a diminished view of health care because it limits the opportunity for the person to find meaning in the health event and learn from or grow through the experience. Unfortunately, the health-care system is organised from a medical model stance which may make it difficult to assert a holistic perspective.

From a holistic perspective, nursing is the unique human encounter between the practitioner and other person[s], however person is described – whether as patient, relative, client or consumer. This encounter is always unique in the sense that it has never been experienced before, although the nurse may have experienced many similar situations that inform this particular situation. Similarly, theory may inform the nurse of the patient's experience or how best to proceed under specific conditions. However, theory cannot prescribe because of the unique situation. Once a nurse accepts theory as prescriptive, it immediately reduces the situation to an object to be manipulated towards certain ends. The humanness of the situation is constantly denied. The nurse becomes a technician who follows certain rules and in so doing, inevitably denies her own humanness. The nurse's primary responsibility shifts from carrying out the doctor's orders to working with and supporting the patient and family in response to the medical prescription whilst pursuing a complementary nursing agenda.

Human care values in nursing

The idea of holism is expanded through the work of Jean Watson (1988). She states that:

> 'The goal of nursing proposed is to help persons gain a higher degree of harmony within the mind, body, and soul which generates self-knowledge, self-reverence, self-healing, and self-care processes while allowing increasing diversity. This goal is pursued through the human–human caring process and caring transactions that respond to the subjective inner world of the person in such a way that the nurse helps individuals find meaning in their existence, disharmony, suffering, and turmoil and promotes self-control, choice, and self-determination with the health–illness decisions.' (p. 49)

These words may, at first glance, seem very different from the words used to compose the Burford philosophy. Yet Watson's words are the closest philosophical statement I have found to express the underlying assumption of the purpose of nursing as human caring. Savour the words and sense the meaning. Can nursing be defined in this way? The human–human encounter is at the root of her description, whereby the central purpose of nursing is to work with the other to enable them to find meaning in the health event. Watson spirals nursing out of the realm of the medical model into a world of existential suffering where the uniqueness and mystery of what it is to be human is fundamental to healing and fulfilment of human potential. Disease and illness are part of the pattern, although the part that often creates crisis for the person.

Watson's words are offered as a moment for reflection, as a challenge to widen the nurse's vision of what caring might mean, not as a prescription of how the nurse should think about nursing. I know that such statements may seem far removed from the messy daily business of nursing, yet Watson pays explicit attention to this messy world by noting the risks to caring both on an individual and societal level.

> 'Caring values of nurses and nursing have been submerged. Nursing and society are, therefore, in a critical situation today in sustaining human care ideals and a caring ideology in practice. The human care role is threatened by increased medical technology, bureaucratic-managerial institutional constraints in a nuclear age society. At the same time there has been a proliferation of curing and radical treatment cure techniques often without regard to costs.' (Watson, 1988, p. 33)

Watson's words emphasise the need to pay attention to 'social viability'. Practitioners may think these 'political' issues are above them but unless they accept a responsibility for caring on a societal plane as well as their everyday practice plane, then there is little chance for nursing to become more valued. The caring ideal as love may be scorned when we as nurses are so damaged or wounded that we cannot care or love. Yet compassion is a reflection of love. Roach (1992) describes compassion as:

> '... a way of living born out of an awareness of one's relationship to all living creatures; engendering a response of participation in the experience of another; a sensitivity to the pain and brokenness of the other; a quality of presence which allows one to share with and make room for the other.' (p. 58)

Watson says that it is this love that provides the driving force to care. Simply, without love for the other person, we cannot care because love *is* care. Without doubt, nurses are aching to care. Such ache is like an unfulfilled love ... remaining unfulfilled, it turns like acid to scar and burnout. Without doubt, patients and families need to be loved by nurses. They ache for this love and when they do not receive it, their disenchantment scars. They experience a sense of being uncared for which is life depleting (Halldórs-dóttir, 1996).

If all this is true, and you will know, then we need to find ways in which nurses can know and realise self as caring within everyday practice.

Modes of being with another

Patients and relatives need to feel cared for at a time of high anxiety (Halldórsdóttir 1996). Studies by Reiman (1986), Mayer (1986), Larson (1987) and Halldórsdóttir (1996) are particularly significant in identifying caring and non-caring encounters. Halldórsdóttir worked with groups of patients including those experiencing cancer. Experiences of cancer were characterised by uncertainty, vulnerability, a sense of isolation, discomfort and redefinition. Because patients expect nurses to be caring, non-caring can contribute to suffering. Non-caring was characterised by insensitivity, disinterest, coldness and inhumanity leading to a decreased sense of well-being for the patient.

The value of this research is to draw the practitioner's attention to her 'mode of being' when working with and caring for patients and families and the impact of her caring on the patient's experience of being cared for. Halldórsdóttir described five modes of nurses being with another, along a continuum from life giving to life destroying (Box 1.4). The realisation that

Box 1.4   Modes of being with another (Halldórsdóttir, 1996).

Modes of being with another	Description
Life giving (biogenic)	A mode where one affirms the personhood of the other by connecting with the true centre of the other in a life-giving way. It relieves the vulnerability of the other and makes the other stronger and enhances growth, restores, reforms and potentiates learning and healing.
Life sustaining (bioactive)	A mode where one acknowledges the personhood of the other, supports, encourages and reassures the other. It gives security and comfort. It positively affects life in the other.
Life neutral (biopassive)	A mode where one does not affect life in the other.
Life restraining (biostatic)	A mode where one is insensitive or indifferent to the other and detached from the true centre of the other. It causes discouragement and develops uneasiness in the other. It negatively affects existing life in the other.
Life destroying (biocidic)	A mode where one depersonalises the other, destroys life and increases the other's vulnerability. It causes distress and despair and hurts and deforms the other. It is transference of negative energy or darkness.

practitioners, through their attitudes and actions, can be uncaring is a profound issue.

REFLECTIVE EXEMPLAR 1.1 TOM'S STORY

I have told Tom's story before in the context of giving meaning to being a reflective practitioner (Johns, 1998b) but it is useful to tell it again as a prompt to consider my own and the care assistant's mode of being with Tom. The story was constructed from my reflective journal after working a shift one day in a community hospital.

I went with Marie, a health-care assistant (HCA), to wash Mr Sturch. I said 'Hello Mr Sturch . . .' and explained who I was. He replied 'Call me Tom'. I immediately sensed his need to be recognised and respected for who he was together with his need for familiarity. We had been informed at the handover of how miserable Tom was being in hospital and being shut in a single room because of the risk of cross infection due to his diarrhoea. We were waiting for results of a bowel culture. If Tom's stool became at least semi-solid, he could be moved back into the main ward.

As I was scheduled to work with Marie, I paid attention to who she was. She was in her fifties and very committed to caring. She loved it and would love to be a nurse. She was experiencing some strain in her personal life, with her mother very ill. She and her husband had moved here some years ago. Now she was having to spend every weekend driving about three hours each way to care for her mother. I listened and was sensitive to being available to her and helped her talk through her options, even though she had not met me before.

Marie's approach to Tom was familiar and, caring but task focused. I immediately noted the characteristic pattern of parent–child communication. Tom was like a little boy, upset but trying hard to be good. Mother was protective, kind, although her tolerance was limited to the extent that there was work to be done. I asked Tom how he felt this morning. He easily expressed his distress at being in hospital and shut up in this room. His tears were close to the surface. He felt lonely shut inside a side room and embarrassed he had diarrhoea that these poor girls had to clean up. Marie kindly informed him that we were going to wash him. This was not negotiated with him. He needed considerable physical help as he had Parkinson's disease. His left hand in particular continued to tremor and. his right side was weakened by a previous stroke.

We began to wash him as he lay on the bed when he asked for the commode. I noted the impact of his Menière's disease characterised by his nausea on standing. This symptom was poorly controlled. Ensuring he felt safe, we left him to use the commode.

Afterwards we helped him to complete his wash whilst sitting on the commode. I helped him stand whilst Marie wiped his bottom. On seeing Tom like that I was struck by Mary Madrid's (1990) account about the nurse imagining who the patient is in terms of his past. Tom told me that he had been a staff sergeant in the army during the Second World War, working in recruitment training. I imagined him like that. How straight and proud he must have been and now, what a different way to parade. And yet I could say that to him with humour, acknowledging his past while being empathic with this moment. I realised the significance of this approach in respecting people. He had also been an engineer in microwaves, work that reflected his intelligence. I resisted a sense of pity at his current state. Instead I felt a wave of compassion towards him. I had learnt through previous experiences about acknowledging self-discomfort towards patients or families and confronting this through enabling the other to talk through their experience. In this way I converted negative energy (pity) into positive energy (compassion). Stephen Levine (1986) had helped me understand the tension between pity and compassion. He states:

> 'When you are motivated by pity, you are motivated by a dense self-interest. When you are motivated by pity, you are acting on the aversion you have to experiencing someone else's predicament. You want to alleviate their discomfort as a means of alleviating your own. When love touches the pain of the other it is called compassion – whatever the other is experiencing you have room for it in your heart.' (p. 168)

After his wash, Tom cleaned his own teeth. He usually had an electric razor shave because the nurses felt clumsy with wet shaves. Tom liked a wet shave and I was able to do this little thing for him. I was reminded of the title of Martha Macleod's (1994) paper 'It's the little things that count: the hidden complexity of everyday clinical nursing practice' and how this 'little thing' of shaving Tom made a difference in caring. I knew this informed Tom of my concern for him and by paying this attention, my concern was fed and grew. I experienced a mutuality in his response. He began to care for me.

Although we had only just met, I had been involved with him in intimate physical care – washing him, being here while he was on the toilet, wiping his bottom, shaving him – and emotional presence. He easily disclosed other aspects of his life. He had been married for 59 years – to 'wifie', his endearing term for his wife. Indeed, his diamond anniversary was in February. He came alive when talking about his wife and their life. She visited in the afternoons. He desperately wanted to go home but he was anxious about the future. He was so dependent physically and even though they had a support package, he feared he would be too much of a burden. I wondered if he would be happier with television, music or a paper. No, he just wanted 'wifie' and to go home. I was conscious of my need to 'fix it' for him, an almost overwhelming need to take his distress away from him. But of course, I was becoming anxious on his behalf, beginning to absorb his distress which I recognised and could repattern to remain available to him.

He loved his shave. His happiness was for me to take 'Murray mints', his gift in return for my attention, my respect and kindness. In seeking to connect with me, he needed to give me something back. By accepting, I could honour this need and he could honour himself. We began to tune into a reciprocal relationship, where I could respond with an appropriate level of involvement with Tom. In this way I synchronised our rhythms of relating with each other at this moment. In tune with him, I was most available to him.

I was conscious of the ways I paid attention to him in response to his feelings and needs, which had made him so happy that morning when he had been so miserable. Nurses are focused on the tasks of the morning and don't necessarily see him from his perspective. They may see him as a person but that's not their frame for responding. Marie noted the difference in him and passed this off as 'male company being good for him'.

I was able to say when his doctor visited, that Tom's stool was semi-formed and to assert Tom's desire to move into the ward. This request was granted. I could also challenge the inadequacy of the medical treatment of his Menière's symptom, to prompt a review of the medical response. The doctor welcomed my feedback. I felt good. I also had several sweets that morning.

Commentary

Perhaps Marie's mode of being was life restraining yet she would have been horrified to view herself as such. Her response to Tom had become routinised and as a consequence his care had been depersonalised, focused around maintaining his physical needs. In contrast, my own mode of being was life giving, connecting with him at the core of his own concerns and affirming his personhood.

Now consider each of these five modes of being with another in the context of your own practice. Halldórsdóttir's work provides a powerful lens for viewing self as caring.

All persons are seen and responded to as unitary human beings

The notion of personhood can be further extended by considering the work of Martha Rogers (1986), who pioneered a radical view of nursing that shifted its focus from the reductionist shadow of deficit models of illness to enabling people to learn through health crises and realise their human potential.

Rogers described human beings as *unitary*. By this, she meant that human beings cannot be reduced to parts without losing their humanness. People need to be responded to as a *whole* in terms of both the meaning that this health event experience has for them and those who are part of their environment, most notably the family network.

Within a holistic caring model, the practitioner views the person/family primarily in terms of the meaning[s] the person gives to their health/illness experience. This understanding is essential in knowing how best to respond to the person/family in order to meet the person's health needs. The 'diagnosis' is clearly a significant event because it is often for this reason that the person and family enter your health-care environment. However, for some health-care workers, such as midwives and health visitors, the focus for connection is normal events such as having a child or child development. Yet even in these normal living activities, the hand of medicalisation stretches out to create a potential world of ill health.

To reiterate, the diagnosis is only part of the whole experience of this person's life/health. In Tom's story, his needs were clearly not being met. The nurses' viewing lens was controlled by a medical gaze that obscured a clear vision of his needs. I wrote in my reflective journal – *why are we so blind to the patient's experience?* I have often used my experience with Tom to prompt discussion. The story evokes much passion, guilt and outrage. Yet these same nurses who express such strong emotion seem to be chained by their inappropriate models, seemingly unable to break free although they know there are more congruent ways of responding to clinical practice. It is as though nurses have no control over their professional integrity. They live incongruent lives where the illusions of being caring persons barely paper over the cracks. In time, people who live incongruent lives become alienated from self in the struggle to maintain the facade. As Jourard (1971) informs us, people alienated from self are unable to be with and care for others. Caring becomes perfunctory. Blindness is the refuge of those in despair, preventing them from seeing the truth.

Rogers further considered the essential nature of humanness; human beings are energy fields that exist beyond the physical body and integrate with environmental energy fields. As such, people affect and are affected by their environments. This has important implications for enabling people to lead healthy lives in caring environments. From this perspective the practitioner becomes part of the environmental field of the patient and vice versa; the way the patient perceives the practitioner and the health-care environment impacts greatly on them and vice versa. Of course, the nurse is also human and *who she is* is central to the care she offers in working with the person and family requiring assistance to meet their health needs. Consider the way Tom perceived and interacted with Marie and myself as part of his environment.

Rogers also considered that people are always in the process of dynamic change, always evolving and becoming more complex. She identified a perspective shift from homoeostasis to homoeodynamics where the intent of health care and nursing is not to return people to previous states but to enable people to grow through the health-care experience. This growth includes the practitioner because the health-care encounter is a mutual process. Each caring encounter is an opportunity for the practitioner's own growth. Reflection gives the practitioner access to this growth opportunity, as evidenced in Tom's story. Tom's story becomes my story of learning through this encounter with him.

Rogers highlighted that each encounter is unpredictable and non-repeating. As such, it is not possible for the practitioner to accurately gauge either the meaning or response before the event; there is always a process of interpretation within the event. Of course, the practitioner has experience of many similar events and theoretical knowledge which informs her within the situation yet the risk of this is that she will impose meaning rather than understand the person's unique meaning and respond appropriately. Thus caring must begin with this recognition – 'who is this (unique evolving) person?'. The person is viewed in terms of the meaning this event has for him in the context of all people and things that matter. From this perspective, I viewed Tom in the moment yet in anticipation of a future as yet unpredictable.

The intent of nursing is to enable the other to realise recovery and growth as expanding consciousness through appropriate caring-healing responses

Another way to view my work with Tom is to see his present and his future as unfolding possibilities, a potential for his growth and fulfilment or what Newman (1994) describes as expanded consciousness. Tom was in crisis, yet the crisis presented an opportunity to search and find meaning in life. My role as a nurse was to help him and his wife reflect and learn through their experience towards self-realisation. As Newman notes:

> 'The new paradigm of health, essential to nursing, embraces a unitary pattern of changing relationships. It is developmental. The task is not to try to change another person's pattern but to recognise it as information that depicts the whole and relate to it as it unfolds.' (p. 13)

Newman expanded a view of health care beyond the medical model's focus on disease and health deficit. Disease confronts the often taken for granted nature of health and prompts a crisis within that person's life. The crisis can be read as a pattern by the practitioner who recognises and explores the signs that lead to deeper underlying factors of which the patient or family may be unaware. Newman was inspired and influenced by the work of Rogers and other theorists whose ideas she integrated within her vision of nursing as 'health as expanding consciousness'. Elements of this influence are set out in Box 1.5 with my interpretation of its significance in the context of the Burford model.

Box 1.5   Key influences within Newman's theory of 'health as expanding consciousness' (1994).

> *Prigogine (1980) Theory of dissipative structures*
> People present in crisis at certain times in their lives when the existing order of things breaks down. The nurse works with the person to help the other learn through the crisis to reorganise self to emerge at a higher level of consciousness.
>
> *Bohm (1980) Theory of implicate order*
> Who people are (the *explicate order*) can be read as a pattern that ripples across the surface of their being. This gives signs and pathways to the deeper self (the *implicate order*) that lies beneath the surface. To help the other, the nurse must appraise this pattern.
>
> *Young (1976) Theory of evolutionary consciousness*
> People need to find meaning in events in order to make good decisions about their lives. This requires the person to know self and become unbound from previous ways that constrain self in order to take necessary action along a pathway of becoming and transformation.

Newman commented that to view the world from a different perspective, requires a paradigm shift which *incorporates the old paradigm and transforms it* (p. 13). In transcending our own boundaries as nurses, we have to move beyond and embrace new ideas and new language. Because we probe things with our minds rather than embracing things with our hearts, we tend to reject certain ideas that are framed in complex language. If we aspire to be holistic then such descriptions challenge us to move beyond our own limited conceptualisations. This is why it is imperative that practitioners begin with their own conceptualisations using their own language. Only by being rooted in our strong beliefs can we engage the philosophy of others.

Prigogine's theory of dissipative structures

I visualised Tom in crisis prompted by a breakdown in predictable health patterns. The breakdown is experienced as a period of disorganisation, unpredictability and uncertainty. Events are experienced as chaotic. The person feels unable to respond adequately to the unfolding events. From this perspective, the event is threatening. To survive, the natural response is to defend self, drawing on learnt defence systems that are themselves incapacitating. I guide Tom and his wife through the crisis to find order within the apparent chaos, to emerge literally on a higher plane of being, or *expanded consciousness*, to become more fulfilled as a human being. The holistic practitioner, in working with the person and family, creates a safer place for the person to be open to the experience and explore the meaning of the health event. Such events are always unpredictable simply because they have not been experienced before.

Bohm's theory of implicate order

I read Tom's pattern for signs to the deeper self in order to enable him to find meaning in his health experience and to *know him from* a holistic perspective. Rogers described nursing assessment as *pattern appreciation appraisal* (Cowling, 1990), refering to the practitioner reading and interpreting this 'pattern'. My response is aimed at *deliberative mutual patterning* whereby I work with Tom to pattern his and his wife's environmental field to promote harmony (Barrett, 1990). *Harmony* is a dynamic yet stable process of evolution. By delving within the implicate order, the person can be helped to see how life patterns have manifested in disorder or crisis. Tom and his wife can then be helped to repattern their lives to find harmony and control in order to respond to future events. Working with the person to understand the meaning of the health event for them will lead to a consideration of all aspects of the person's life but not as a haphazard and intrusive action.

Young's theory of evolutionary consciousness

I enabled Tom to talk about his life and health issues to help him recognise and feel empowered to make the right choices, difficult as some of these choices might be because he does not feel empowered or because of the potential consequences. This process means being there for the person to inform, advise, help the person make sense of and support them with these choices. It also means confronting them when these choices seem inappropriate or when the person cannot see beyond the barriers that limit potential. The nurse responds appropriately to release the healing energy within the other person through empathy and love (Moss, 1981). Moss argues that expanding consciousness is always a mutual process because in giving self to the other, self must inevitably be fulfilled in realising its therapeutic potential. Through reflection, this realisation can be acknowledged and honoured.

The poem 'Nursing as expanded consciousness' captures the parallel healing space of clinical practice and guided reflection. As you read the poem, reflect on the ideas within Newman's work and the way these ideas fuse reflective and caring theory. Within the poem, the tipi is a metaphor for a quiet place for reflection.

Nursing as expanded consciousness

The tipi is both a sacred and safe place.
It is sacred space because it is who I am,
And who I am and who you are
Form the caring dance.
It is a safe place because I wrap myself in who a nurse is,
To protect me from the storms and from the blistering sun,
Symbols for the deep distress of your suffering.

Sacred and safe,
To find rhythm and harmony in the caring dance.
Through reflection I can find and know who I am.
I can tune the caring dance;
In harmony with you
I am available to you.

The dance is working with you
And with your kindred,
To help you find meaning in this experience,
To enable you to make best decisions about your life
So you are empowered to take action,
So you can emerge through the crisis
On a higher level of consciousness
In harmony with self and others.

I read the pattern that ripples across your being;
Signs that lead us to visit the deeper parts
Where healing can take place;
I tune into who you are,
To ride your wavelength in synchrony,
Surfing the tides of emotion
As you fluctuate with the unfolding moments
A shelter from the storms and the blistering sun,
A playground to laugh and play,
A soul friend along the way.

The caring dance....
I reflect within the moment
To stay in tune with you;
I hold the mirror to reflect on
This experience with you
In words that spill across my journal's pages.

Sometimes it is not easy to see self,
And to see beyond self.
It helps when another holds the mirror for me,
To help me find meaning in my experience,
To enable me to make good decisions about my practice
So I am empowered to take appropriate action;
To tame the demons of contradiction that bind me tight,
To nurture my concern for you
Often at a time of crisis
When I might rather hide within the tipi's shadows.

Learning through the experience I honour myself
I pay tribute to my sacred self
I can open the tipi for all to see
So I too can emerge at a higher level of consciousness;
Nourished in the orange glow;
Connecting caring and being cared for,
Rhythms in harmony.

As a carer I am not alone;
Through caring I am connected across the globe,
Connected through the cosmos blue
That encircles us – as here today.
We expand ever outwards;
Nursing as expanded consciousness
Reaching to fulfil our caring destiny.

Christopher Johns (1998)

Chapter 2

Establishing a Reflective Dialogue with the Patient

From beliefs to practice

Writing a philosophy is a creative moment that gives practitioners a collective voice to articulate the meaning of their practice. Yet how can a philosophy become a lived reality? Rawnsley (1990) offers a profound challenge.

> 'Caring may be a desirable image for nursing, but is it meaningful? Is there congruence between the lived experience of nursing practice and the intellectual pursuit of caring as nursing's professional crest? When living the reality of their practice, nurses need ways through which they can connect the conceptual concerns of the discipline with the raw data of experience.' (p. 42, cited in Johns, 1994, p. 6)

Consider to what extent is your own philosophy a reality within practice. What factors limit this achievement? Just because practitioners think and feel about nursing from a holistic perspective does not mean they can achieve this in practice. I am sure all practitioners can identify many situations of contradiction between what they wanted to achieve in working with a patient and actual practice. I am also sure that many nurses go home each day with this sense of contradiction. It manifests itself as a disquiet, a sense of dissatisfaction, anger or even guilt.

An expanded view of the whole model

Box 2.1 sets out the overall structure for a reflective model for (nursing) practice.

At the centre of this model is the philosophy for practice. Four reflective systems of connection are proposed to enable practitioners to effectively realise the philosophy as everyday practice.

(1) A system for operationalising the philosophy within each unfolding moment
(2) A system for ensuring effective communication
(3) A system for ensuring staff are developed to use the model in effective ways
(4) A system to ensure the model realises effective practice

Box 2.1   Structural view of the Burford model.

A culture that enhances clinical leadership	*A system for ensuring effective communication*	A culture of clearly defined role responsibility and collaborative teamwork
A system for operationalising the philosophy within each unfolding moment	Practitioner[s] belief system (expressed as a *valid* philosophy of care)	*A system for ensuring staff are developed to use the model in effective ways*
A culture for creativity and positive risk management	*A system to ensure the model realises effective practice*	A culture that values holistic practice

A system for operationalising the philosophy within each unfolding moment

How can a practitioner be guided to reflect on and respond to each clinical moment in tune with the hospital philosophy? It is proposed that a reflective model consists of a series of reflective cues to tune the practitioner into the caring concepts within the philosophy as a continuous process of grasping and interpreting the situation, envisaging what needs to be achieved, responding appropriately with effective action and evaluating and reflecting on the consequences.

A system for ensuring effective communication

How can a practitioner communicate effectively to ensure the patient and the family receive consistent and congruent care from all health-care workers? Is the nursing process an adequate method to achieve this or are there more meaningful and practical ways for both verbal and written reflection and communication?

A system for ensuring staff are developed to use the model in effective ways

How can a practitioner develop her ability to be an effective holistic and reflective practitioner? The advent of guided reflection or clinical supervision offers an opportunity to learn through experience to develop and sustain effective practice.

A system to ensure the model realises effective practice

How can practitioners get valid feedback that practice is making a significant difference to the health care of patients and families? One way is through guided reflection. More formal ways are through reflective reviews and the development of reflective standards of care that allow practitioners to accept responsibility for ensuring the development and efficacy of aspects of clinical practice.

Cultural accommodation

Each of these four systems is unfolded through the book. Being reflective, each of these systems is sensitive to feedback in order to ensure their continuous integrated development and efficacy. However, it is imperative to acknowledge that structures alone will not lead to effective holistic practice. Holistic practice is a deeply human encounter between people. Structures merely create opportunity through which caring and change processes can be guided.

To accommodate reflective practice or indeed any radical change within practice, it is necessary to foster certain cultural conditions (as set out in the four corners of Box 2.1). Understanding the way these cultural conditions support a culture of reflective practice acknowledges that managing change is a social process that will inevitably challenge deeply embedded norms. These four cultural conditions are visible just below the surface of all discussion and stories within the book. Sometimes the influence of these conditions is made explicit and sometimes it is understated. As such, a brief synopsis of each condition may be helpful.

A culture that enhances clinical leadership

Chapter 1 has highlighted the leadership role of establishing a shared vision for practice that sets up the necessary developmental processes to realise the philosophy as an everyday reality. Perhaps most significantly, leadership is concerned with driving and managing change as a social process that acknowledges, understands and brings people together to resolve the cultural shifts required to accommodate effective holistic and reflective practice.

A culture of clearly defined role responsibility and collaborative teamwork

The very nature of holism is grounded in working with colleagues in mutual *responsible* ways within clearly identified roles. A holistic model for organising care must acknowledge the value of each person and emphasise mutual ways of relating and supporting the common philosophy to realise caring in practice. This necessarily means confronting existing relational patterns that constrain collaborative work, most notably patterns that have been constructed through hierarchical ways of relating which have traditionally fostered dependence and subordination in nurses.

A *culture that values holistic practice*

Reflective practice is symbiotic with a holistic approach to health care. As such, it will flourish in a culture that values holistic caring practices and practitioners. Unfortunately the prevailing culture of health-care organisations does not seem to value caring beyond the rhetoric. If this is true then nurses need always to assert caring against a gradient of disinterest. To do so effectively, the reflective practitioner becomes a political operator in confronting the organisation with the contradictions between its rhetoric and its practice. Not easy work if it is also true that nurses perceive themselves as subordinate and powerless (Buckenham & McGrath, 1983).

I have already noted the empowering impact of constructing a philosophy as a bottom-up collaborative activity. In doing so, practitioners become active creators of their own practice and take responsibility for realising their beliefs within practice. This means confronting those who wish to keep nursing in the shadow of organisational and medical dominance. Perhaps in the face of such social reality it is easier to live out the illusion and pretend to ourselves we are holistic rather than confront the status quo and act from integrity. Perhaps when nurses reflect on how patients suffer through neglect of caring then they will become empowered to confront, understand and learn through the contradiction between their holistic-based beliefs and the way they actually practise. This inevitably means confronting the organisational conditions of practice.

A *culture for creativity and positive risk management*

NHS Trusts are conscious of public image and litigation. Indeed, a cynical view might be that NHS Trusts are more concerned with public image than with patient care. Nurses are in an unenviable firing line between management and the patient/family. Patient and family anxiety is projected onto nurses, as is management anxiety. Nurses have internalised this anxiety by becoming consciously concerned with managing potential complaints (Johns, 1995a). This projection of anxiety often results in nurses becoming the scapegoat for events. Such a climate leads nurses to be defensive rather than creative with the consequence that they do not feel in control of their own practice and feel powerless to implement change. A reflective practice perspective offers a positive approach to learning through the complaint experience.

Reflect on each factor within Box 2.1. Do you work in a culture that will facilitate reflective practice? Do not despair if you are not optimistic. As I shall discuss, the first step in becoming a reflective practitioner is to become open and curious about your practice. 'Why are things as they are?' 'How might they be different to help us realise our philosophy as a lived reality?' We need to understand the way things are as a precursor to changing practice.

Establishing the reflective dialogue with the patient

As we begin to consider how caring beliefs can become a lived reality through reflective practice, our attention must first be focused on the relationship between the practitioner and the person and family who seek help in response to some health event. Johns (1994) noted:

> 'The prime focus of assessment must be to recognise and respond to the humanness of the patient in order to establish a working and caring relationship, or what Paterson and Zderad (1988, p. 23) describe as a "lived dialogue".' (p. 41)

Drew (1986) categorised people's experience of care (on surgical units) as essentially one of exclusion or confirmation. Drew noted:

> 'A first step towards the humanisation of health care is the explication of the experience of patients with caregivers and the meanings that those patients attributed to their encounters with them.' (p. 43)

Given that human beings are self-determining, the practitioner must establish a reflective dialogue to understand the other's experience, with the intention of helping them find meaning in their health experience and enabling them to make the best decisions about their health care. Gadow (1980) describes such dialogue as *existential advocacy*, which means *being within* the unfolding moment to work with the other 'whole' person and family to help them to find meaning in their experience. The practitioner tunes into the pattern of the other, to literally get onto their wavelength in order to synchronise self with the other to establish what I call the 'caring dance'.

Reflective cues

Knowing the person is fundamental to establishing the existential dialogue. I view and respond to each clinical situation through a *reflective* lens which consists of nine reflective cues, each of which has been constructed to tune the practitioner into the caring concepts that comprise the philosophy of the Burford NDU model. The reflective practitioner internalises these cues (Box 2.2) as a *natural* way of seeing and responding appropriately within each unfolding clinical moment; she does not give the cues conscious thought as she approaches each patient or family member. Yet, as a reflective practitioner, I constantly test the continued appropriateness of these cues to guide my caring practice. (The cues are explored in depth in Chapter 4.)

These cues help me to tune into the other person and to read the pattern of signs that reveal the deeper self of the patient and myself (Newman, 1994). Read again Tom's story in Chapter 1 – and sense the way these cues guided me to see and respond to Tom.

Box 2.2 The Burford NDU model reflective cues.

Core question: What information do I need to be able to nurse this person?

Cue questions

- Who is this person?
- What meaning does this illness/health event have for the person?
- How is this person feeling?
- How has this event affected their usual life patterns and roles?
- How do I feel about this person?
- How can I help this person?
- What is important for this person to make their stay in hospital comfortable?
- What support does this person have in life?
- How does this person view the future for themselves and others?

REFLECTIVE EXEMPLAR 2.1: HELEN AND KIM

Consider the way Helen established an existential relationship with Kim through the reflective cues. Helen is a clinical nurse specialist (CNS) in nutrition. The dialogue has been constructed from notes recorded during a guided reflection session between Helen and myself (the nature of guided reflection is explored in Chapter 3). Helen had drafted her revised philosophy for practice constructed within the principles of the Burford NDU model philosophy (Box 2.3).

Helen: "Using the Burford model has confronted me with the fact that people have real feelings. It has provoked a chain of thinking – 'why do I go to visit these patients?' I got a feeling of not offering them anything except maybe to increase their safety. I am actively making this effort to see them as people – to see them differently from how I have been."
CJ: "Does this lead to increased satisfaction?"
Helen: "Yes, although it makes it tougher, but in a sense it has challenged my 'task' approach. Now, I probably see fewer patients in a day. That in itself is frustrating but I am more satisfied with what I do."
CJ: "A key aspect of your work is managing priorities and time?"
Helen: "It is the crux of the clinical nurse specialist's role. I don't want to 'police' others' work but that's what I had become. At least the danger of it, if that hasn't totally happened. It may also be a problem of being part-time – I don't work enough hours. Maybe I need to work more hours or maybe it's a problem of the way I work – the 'beat the clock thing'. The reflective cues – 'How must this person be feeling?' and 'How do I feel about this person?' keep popping into my head. I had a situation with a patient, Kim – it changed the whole way the experience went. She is 26 with Crohn's disease. She has a nasty fistula pouring fluid. She is on total parenteral

Box 2.3   Helen's philosophy of care

I believe . . .

- That nursing care offered by the CNS nutrition is centred around the needs of the patient. To this end, the CNS will be available to teach and support patients receiving nutritional support, which will enable them to become partners in their own care. Care is extended to the patient's family and friends as desired.

- That care should be holistic in nature, whether towards recovery through the use of aggressive nutritional support or towards adaptation with altered health states, including death. At all times, the patient's safety and comfort are paramount. The patient's right to confidentiality and privacy will be respected.

- That when nutritional support is continued after discharge from hospital, the CNS will ensure the provision of seamless care. To this end, the patient discharged on nutritional support will have received adequate teaching and equipment and will feel supported by the CNS, in association with other health-care workers, until they become confident to continue independently.

- That the CNS may act as primary carer or role model and teacher of nurses and other carers. In so doing the CNS will strive to continually improve patient care, by implementing appropriate research findings and by ongoing evaluation of care. This develops the social value of nursing, and enables others to benefit from the CNS's expertise.

- That in order to be effective, the CNS will need to manage conflict and so will share her feelings openly at appropriate times. She will support others when needed, reciprocating the caring approach to patients.

nutrition (TPN). I visited her on the ward. Her dressing had been done. The Hickman line should have been fixed in – she had sat on it and it pulled out. The doctor said he would sort another one but she said 'No!'.

I went in and knew she would not get better without it – my intention was to be forceful just like the doctors. And then I stopped myself – asked myself 'Why am I acting like this?'. I noted my own feelings – that I was anxious she was not safe without the TPN. I asked how was she feeling. She was reacting against having the TPN forced on her. She has been like this for two years, her life has been turned upside down with no feeling of control – her only control was to say 'No!'. I confronted her with this – 'Is this how you are feeling?'. She said 'Yes!! That's exactly how I am feeling. I am not having it'. I sat and talked it through with her. In the end we negotiated a compromise: that she could go home for the weekend to spend it with her children without the line and return on Monday to have the line resited. We agreed!"

CJ: "You saw the person instead of the problem?"

Helen: "It was wonderful. I went home beaming! Since then I have had other situations with doctors rushing her. For example, her Hb was 6.7 and she needed a blood transfusion. She told them to 'push off!' saying 'I'm an honorary Jehovah's Witness'. But give her time and she will mull it over. Eventually she said she was happy with this. When they put the second line in the intention was to put two units of blood through it before the TPN. I said to the consultant on the round 'No. That's for the TPN'. I confronted him. He agreed with me. But 2–3 weeks later the doctors tried to give her another transfusion through the 'Cuff Cath'. She said to them 'No you're not, Helen said no'. The doctor went to the consultant who agreed with me that they were not doing that. I had told Kim why it was important, that it contaminated the line with the risk of CVP sepsis."

Commentary

The Burford reflective cues triggered Helen to see Kim behind the medical label. Previously Helen had essentially viewed the patient through a medical-oriented lens that had encouraged her to focus on the organ dysfunction and, more specifically, on the nutritional consequences. Kim was no longer a 'problem' to solve but a person whose anxieties and suffering were responded to within the existential dialogue. Helen enabled Kim's voice to be heard – her cry of rebellion and anguish against being manipulated as an object. By listening to Kim, Helen enhanced the medical treatment. Caring incorporates and transcends the technical task. Once Helen had accepted Kim's perspective, her own anxiety melted away. The outcome was empowering for herself and Kim. Caring had been realised and its value reinforced.

REFLECTIVE EXEMPLAR 2.2: TONY'S STORY

Consider my effort to establish an existential dialogue with Tony. The account is taken from my reflective journal after working at the hospice one day – I was working with Susan on the 'shop floor'. We started by helping Alice, a woman who required some assistance to wash. She was happy for me to help her, although I was sensitive to any sense of intrusion and embarrassment on her behalf. Would a woman who was terminally ill like to be helped to wash by a strange man? However, I didn't sense any resistance. Nurses can be insensitive to patients requiring intimate care. They take it for granted that patients will accept being nursed by any nurse, male or female. This seemed more taken for granted by female nurses because of the stereotypical societal role of women as carers. In considering the Burford NDU model cues – 'who is this person?' and 'what is important to make this person's stay in hospital comfortable?', the practitioner develops a sensitivity towards the sexuality of the patient.

I then went to help Tony get up for lunch. He is 53 and has primary lung cancer with liver secondaries. He is in the hospice for respite care. He has been here just four days and he wants to go home. In his words, 'Not that it's unpleasant in here but...' Unspoken words but I sensed he didn't like the reminder of his forthcoming death. There were cards on the wall made by his grand-daughter. He could talk about her and I could tell she was very special to him, perhaps adding to his sense of sadness. Things that make us happy also make us sad – the Heideggerian notion that we choose to pay attention to things because they matter to us. As Benner & Wrubel (1989) note, the things that do matter to us are the things that make us vulnerable, two sides of the same coin. This is the same for the nurse. In opening myself to being vulnerable, I also seek ways in which I can manage my vulnerability yet without diminishing my sense of concern. This is both internal – knowing 'who I am' and managing my inter-relationship with others within the context of what is desirable – and external – establishing a caring environment in which I work to balance my caring with others.

So as I gazed at Tony, I sensed that his life was a constant search for balance at the edge of chaos. I was conscious of my need to tune into this balance without being intrusive. I sensed his irritation with me. Did he want me to go? Should I accept his dismissal of me or assert my authority to be his helper whether he liked it or not? To be a *good patient*, he should conform to my presence – an ironic twist! But what potential anarchy if we accepted that all patients had the right to choose whom they should be nursed by?

So, I hung around him, trying hard to be available to help him if he wanted it. I had been told that he struggled to co-ordinate himself, perhaps his dexamethasone was affecting him. He needed but didn't want my help. I picked up this ambivalence and felt uncomfortable, not wanting to irritate him but recognising that he would need some help. I was trying hard to keep a positive space in which to work together yet it was difficult tuning in and remaining on his wavelength. Perhaps he wanted Susan, whom he knew and felt comfortable with. Yet, being a good patient, he couldn't tell me that ... at least in words.

Tony got himself into the shower and eventually dressed. This took about an hour. His pain was well controlled. In writing that, I confront myself – why are nurses so focused on pain? Perhaps *we* understand, feel comfortable with and feel more useful with such concrete issues as symptom management than responding meaningfully to his sense of irritation. We talked about schooling, my children and his grand-daughter. He had been a plumber; he knew he was not going back to work any more and accepted that. He remained superficially accepting of my presence but I sensed that his irritation continued to ripple over him. I was tempted to let him know that I sensed this, to ask if I was bothering him. This confrontation might prick the tension, yet it might also embarrass him.

I decided to pick up the cue of his discomfort at being in the hospice. This was his major irritation, I merely exacerbated it. I acknowledged that he needed to go home, feeding back my understanding and acceptance of this need. I felt my continual anxiety. I never felt comfortable with him but then why should I? And why shouldn't he be irritated? He seemed to relax more when he discovered I was an academic, as if he could then accept my being here more easily, rather than some new nurse he had never met before and the need to decide whether to go through it all again – the effort of making a relationship. He was intrigued by my academic role at the hospice. This was an important understanding – that he needed to know me, to put me into context in order to accept my presence more than simply as 'a visiting nurse'. Even though that was true, it was a conservative truth. Why should he be pestered by an inquisitive visiting nurse when he was confronting his own death and the loss of his relationship with his grand-daughter? For whose benefit was the pestering? Could I pretend to be helping him? Does the need to be useful or, even worse, to fix it for him become a mentality that reduces Tony to some curious object?

We got to lunch . . . everybody else had gone. I stayed with him until he had finished. By then I had tuned into him and felt at ease with him. There is something normalising about having a chat outside the immediate care environment and having a meal with someone. He had been a keen cyclist which gave us something concrete and interesting to talk about.

On reflection, it had been an apparently uncomfortable 90 minutes where I struggled to manage my ambivalent feelings towards this man, even as he struggled to manage his ambivalent feelings towards me. It highlighted for me the fundamental need to know people in order to respond appropriately to them on a level that is meaningful and non-intrusive. This requires a deep concern and a mutuality. We were getting there but it required an immense effort. Should I have bothered or simply said to Susan 'this man needs you'? This is also a profound understanding because nurses need to recognise that they are not omnipotent and cannot help everybody all the time. Whilst I could connect superficially by helping him wash and dress, escort him to his lunch, monitor and administer his pain and other symptom relief, this was not the level of help he really needed. On a deeper level he was in spiritual crisis. I could read that but that was my difficulty. I could not respond easily to the superficial caring issues outside that deeper context. Hence helping him wash and dress became difficult once I had looked into his eyes and felt the pain. He also knew that, which made it difficult for him. Perhaps he would have preferred the nurse going superficially about her business, barely touching the surface of his deeper concerns. Perhaps I simply needed to be available to him so he could use me if he needed to do so. Over time he could make this decision based on knowing who I was. As it was, on this first encounter, I felt intrusive, as if my need to be caring trapped me.

Later I shared this experience with Susan. She affirmed my experience, acknowledging Tony's struggle in facing his death. She also acknowledged my difficulty in tuning into him, but felt I shouldn't worry unduly about that. Susan acknowledged that Tony was 'difficult' and, *ipso facto*, that my experience was normal, the flattening of sensitivity in order to cope with the stresses of the day. Yet Susan's concern for me was genuine.

Writing has helped me work through some issues that I had been conscious of within the moment but which have become clearer. Now, I feel positive towards Tony. My compassion has been fed and has grown. I feel no sense of pity towards him despite his deep sense of impending loss. Indeed, I look forward to picking up my relationship with him.

My effort was to establish the existential dialogue with Tony, grounded in helping him find meaning in his experience. Tony is in crisis – this crisis ripples across his being to be read and responded to. Yet how do I respond appropriately to a stranger as he faces his own death and the impending loss of his grand-daughter? Am I sensitive enough? Do I intrude? Should I withdraw? Why am I so concerned about this experience? Therein lies my skill as a holistic practitioner – to make such judgements. There is no pre-scription, there is only the judgement within the unfolding moment of the caring dance.

I became part of Tony's environmental field just as he became part of mine. My intent was to tune into his rhythm, to get onto Tony's wavelength. The person receiving care will acknowledge this synchronicity – 'this nurse understands me, this nurse is concerned for me'. We begin the caring dance. Through the continuous dialogue this rhythm or pattern of relating is developed. In doing so, meaning is constantly being reconstructed. If Tony wants to keep me at a distance then I understand this and tune into him at this distance, yet still communicating my concern for him. He reads my pattern and invites me closer. I monitor and manage my own feelings of being rejected by him.

Advocacy

I knew that my therapeutic response was to *be available* to Tony, to help him find meaning and harmony through his experience, to be a sanctuary or soul-level friend (Bolen, 1996) with whom Tony could reflect and grow. My role was not to fix it for him or to take it personally but to hear, accept and to open up a healing space. I could not take away his angst yet I could be a secure place where he could work towards finding meaning in his pain and where he could grow. To achieve this I needed to work to create this space where he could feel cared for enough to share.

Seedhouse (1988) claims that respecting autonomy and creating the opportunity for another to exercise his autonomy are the highest ethical principles. In other words, Tony has the right to self-determination and my duty is to help him exercise this right. After all, it is his life and his death. Health-care practitioners need to be quite clear about their roles in working with patients and families who are often bewildered and unable to make good decisions and need to be dependent on others for a while. The effective practitioner reads this pattern and responds appropriately, accepting the patient's dependence at this moment in time. Tomorrow is a new day and dependence may shift to prompt a new response. Making decisions on behalf of another person is termed *paternalism*, which can be viewed along a therapeutic continuum with advocacy (Box 2.4).

Box 2.4   The advocacy – paternalism therapeutic continuum.

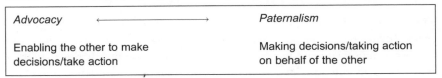

Advocacy ⟵————————⟶	*Paternalism*
Enabling the other to make decisions/take action	Making decisions/taking action on behalf of the other

For paternalism to be therapeutic, i.e. in terms of the patient's or family's best interests, Benjamin & Curtis (1986) claim that three factors need to be justified (Box 2.5).

Box 2.5   Justification criteria of paternalism.

Harm factor	Is the patient likely to come to harm if I don't take action?
Autonomy factor	Is the patient unable to make the decision for himself?
Ratification factor	Would the patient at a later time ratify my decision as being in his best interests?

The dilemma that often faces health-care workers is the individual's right of self-determination measured against the harm factor, balancing one ethical principle (autonomy) against another (beneficence). All health-care workers live out the daily tension of balancing what is therapeutic against what is safe. Perhaps practitioners err on the side of safety for fear of criticism if the people in their care come to some harm. Remember Helen and Kim's story! Then again, Tony might easily have slipped in the shower and hurt himself, yet was staying with him a paternal act or an infringement of his rights? Tony agreed that I should stay, but did he feel obliged to agree? My reflection exposes these dilemmas.

Practitioners who absorb patients' distress and suffering are in danger of responding paternal to protect patients from the seemingly uncaring behaviours of other health-care workers. This interpretation of advocacy is acknowledged by the UKCC Code of Professional Practice clause 1 (1992) which considers advocacy as being concerned with asserting the patient's rights in the face of inhumane health care. However, interpreted in this way, advocacy is perhaps more concerned with nurse empowerment and the management of interpersonal conflict than patient empowerment, although the UKCC emphasises that advocacy is not concerned with conflict for its own sake. The difficulty is that in asserting the rights of patients against the values of dominant others, an issue of interpersonal conflict and power relationships arises rather than an issue about what is best for the patient (Johns, 1996b). Such action is more appropriately described as confrontation; confronting other's restricted beliefs, attitudes or behaviour (Heron, 1975).

The four dialogues of caring

The existential dialogue between Tony and myself is one of four dialogues of caring (Box 2.6). To reiterate, the existential dialogue is the dialogue between the practitioner and the patient or family member in which the patient is affirmed as an individual who determines his own life and death experiences.

Box 2.6   The four dialogues of caring.

- The existential dialogue between the practitioner and the person.
- The dialogue with others in order to synchronise self with other health-care workers to ensure a congruent caring environment.
- The dialogue with self – 'reflection-within-the-moment' to tune into and synchronise self with the person.
- The dialogue with self through use of reflective journalling and/or guided by another to reflect on experience in order to synchronise and reflexively develop the other caring dialogues.

Dialogue with others

Helen's work with Kim illustrates the impact of other health-care workers on their relationship. Helen establishes a reflective dialogue with her colleagues in order to synchronise self with others to ensure that Kim received congruent and consistent care.

Whilst the idea of collaboration to work towards the same goals seems obvious, in reality achieving collaboration is riddled with problems. Practitioners work within the context of finite resources, competing priorities, conflicting values and power relationships that all too often interfere with achieving desirable work and which unfortunately often lead to conflict, frustration and stress and are a threat to caring. This is explored in depth in Chapter 8.

Dialogue with self within the moment

As I listened to Tony and tuned into his wavelength I was constantly processing what he was saying to me, checking out with him if my understanding was correct and my response appropriate. I was also paying attention to the way I felt with Tony drawing on the reflective cue 'How do I feel about this person?'. As the story illuminates, I felt anxious. Hence I had to deal with my anxiety in ways that did not compromise the therapeutic moment and allowed me to remain available to Tony. The ability to manage self within therapeutic relationships is explored in depth in Chapter 7.

The dialogue with self within the unfolding moment is termed reflection-within-the-moment (Johns, 1998b). It is a deep sensitivity to self that ripples along the surface of conscious thought in reponse to the unfolding existential dialogue. Reflection-within-the-moment feels similar to Casement's (1985) idea of the *internal supervisor*, whereby the practitioner (in his case, a psychoanalyst) has a critical conversation with self in order to respond appropriately to patient disclosure. It is asking self – what does Tony mean? Why is he irritated with me? How am I feeling? How do I respond for the best? This depth of self-dialogue, although conscious, is internalised as a natural response structured through the reflective cues (Box 2.2). Reflection-within-the-moment is more than Schön's (1987) concept of *reflection-in-action*, which is a process of paying attention, framing and solving problems as they arise during a situation, a kind of problem solving on the hoof in response to a surprise or breakdown in the smooth running of activity. Presumably if no breakdown occurs, habitual practice proceeds as taken for granted (Johns, 1998b).

Dialogue with self on reflection

Tony's story was written in my reflective journal later the same day. Writing my reflective journal creates a space where I can reflect on the significance of the event, pay attention to and work through my feelings. 'Why did I feel so anxious? Why did I feel uncomfortable? How was Tony really feeling? Did I respond appropriately? 'How else might I have responded?' Writing a journal sensitises self to self and has enabled me to become increasingly sensitive within the moment.

The function of reflection on experience is to develop and synchronise the practitioner's ability to work within the other dialogues of caring. The nature of reflection-on-experience is explored in Chapter 3.

Chapter 3

Being and Becoming a Reflective Practitioner

Introduction

This chapter discusses the significance of reflection as a process to facilitate the development of effective practice by learning through everyday lived experience. For many reasons, reflection may need to be guided by another person (Johns, 1998a).

When I introduced guided reflection at Burford in 1989, Gill (the practitioner) and I met for one hour every two weeks. I asked her to share and reflect on any work experiences she felt were significant in some way. We were not guided by any specific theory, although I had searched the literature for relevant information. My response was to listen carefully and ask sensible questions to enable Gill to develop effective practice. This work became my PhD research study, during which the pattern of dialogue was continuously analysed, enabling meaning to be constructed and a theory of guided reflection to evolve (Johns, 1998a).

Reflection

There are many theoretical expositions of reflection which the interested practitioner can explore (Atkins & Murphy, 1993; Fitzgerald, 1994; Johns, 1998a; Johns & Freshwater, 1998). However, it is sensible not to accept definitions on face value. In a technological culture, practitioners often grasp at theoretical definitions and then struggle to fit the experience to the definition, rather than using the definition creatively to guide reflection.

Reflection is a window through which the practitioner can view and focus self within the context of her own lived experience in ways that enable her to confront, understand and work towards resolving the contradictions within her practice between what is desirable and actual practice. Through the conflict of contradiction, the commitment to realise desirable work and understanding why things are as they are, the practitioner is empowered to take more appropriate action in future situations. Reflection opens the person to herself in order to acknowledge and honour herself. In this way, reflection offers a sacred space for the creativity each new day brings (O'Donohue, 1997) as the practitioner comes to realise her potential to make a significant difference to the lives of patients and families.

Reflection can be viewed as a critical social process moving through stages of enlightenment, empowerment and emancipation (Fay, 1987; see Box 3.1).

Box 3.1   Fay's typology of enlightenment, empowerment and emancipation.

Enlightenment (understanding) – understanding why things have come to be as they are in terms of frustrating self's realisation of desirable practice.

Empowerment – focusing the sense of purpose, felt conflict and fear of negative consequences as necessary to take appropriate action towards changing self and the way things are in order to realise desirable practice.

Emancipation (transformation) – the realisation of self's best interests as a consequence of taking appropriate action.

Fay's work shows reflection as a critical social process of overcoming the forces that prevent nurses fulfilling their therapeutic potential and destiny. Yet this makes sense when considering the current nursing ideology of working with and empowering patients from a holistic perspective. To facilitate empowerment in others, nurses must themselves be empowered or free to take appropriate action in responding to the health-care needs of patients and families. Kieffer (1984) noted that the process of empowerment involved:

'... reconstructing and re-orientating deeply engrained personal systems of social relations. Moreover they confront these tasks in an environment which historically has enforced their political repression, and which continues its active and implicit attempts at subversion of constructive change.' (p. 27)

Whilst Kieffer's words are melodramatic, they do draw the practitioner's attention to those factors that limit or constrain them from realising effective caring within everyday practice. Empowerment is the sense of freedom to do something significant in changing one's life. It is the energy and will to move from passivity, the perception of self as powerless often reflected in uncertainty and aggression, towards becoming assertive, able to take confident action considering self's and others' needs.

Reflection is concerned with the growth of the powerful self whereby the practitioner can understand and take action to reconstitute patterns of relating with more powerful others in ways that enable her to realise desirable and effective practice. As Maxine Greene (1988) noted:

'To become [different] is not simply to will oneself to change. There is the question of being *able* to accomplish what one chooses to do. It is not only a matter of the capacity to choose; it is a matter of the power to act to attain one's purposes. We shall be concerned with intelligent choosing and, yes, humane choosing, as we shall be with the kinds of conditions necessary for empowering persons to act on what they choose.' (p. 3)

I prefer the word *transformation* to emancipation because transformation suggests the practitioner is growing out of their old self. The words of Blackwolf Jones and Jones (1996) offer a perspective.

'It is though we are in a cocoon, within a cocoon, within a cocoon. The more truth we experience, the more we are set free in colourful flight. Always in movement, the different levels of consciousness we experience lead us to the next level. This is how we come to soar. (p. 54)

The truth is knowing self, a truth that is always unfolding and liberating.

The ten Cs of reflection

As a guide to its essential nature, reflection can be viewed as ten Cs of reflection (Box 3.2).

Box 3.2   The ten Cs of reflection.

Commitment – believing that self and practice matter; accepting responsibility for self; the openness, curiosity and willingness to challenge normative ways of responding to situations.

Contradiction – exposing and understanding the contradiction between what is desirable and actual practice.

Conflict – harnessing the energy of conflict within contradiction to become empowered to take appropriate action.

Challenge and support – confronting the practitioner's normative attitudes, beliefs and actions in ways that do not threaten the practitioner.

Catharsis – Working through negative feelings.

Creation – moving beyond self to see and understand new ways of viewing and responding to practice.

Connection – connecting new insights within the real world of practice; appreciating the temporality of experience over time.

Caring – realising desirable practice as everyday reality.

Congruence – reflection as a mirror for caring.

Constructing personal knowing in practice – weaving personal knowing with relevant extant theory in constructing knowledge.

Commitment

In order to reflect, the practitioner needs to be open to self and to pay attention to self's experience (Fay, 1987). The reflective practitioner is open and curious about her practice: 'why are things as they are?', 'could things be done in a better way?'. Rather like Edward Bear coming downstairs bumping on the back of his head, thinking 'there must be a better way', if only he could stop bumping a moment to consider it (Milne, 1926). In a busy world it may be difficult to find this space to stop bumping, to consider more appropriate and less painful ways of doing things. Often, because things have become overly familiar we no longer pay attention to them. O'Donohue (1997) notes:

'People have difficulty awakening to their inner world, especially when their lives become over familiar to them. They find it hard to discover something new, interesting or adventurous in their numbed lives.' (p. 122–3)

O'Donohue suggests that over familiarity leads to complacency. Reflection, by its nature, confronts people with their experience. To pay attention to experience in meaningful ways requires a belief that self and practice matter, otherwise why should I want to pay attention to experience? Attention to self requires the practitioner to value self and self-development in a prevailing culture where self-development is generally viewed as low priority. Without being open, curious and committed, the practitioner may struggle to look in the reflective mirror. Indeed it may be uncomfortable to look at self, especially when the self is riddled with contradiction or where commitment has diminished. Commitment is a reflection that things matter to the practitioner. It is a reflection of caring – because these things matter then the practitioner cares for them, she pays attention to them. Reflection requires the practitioner's commitment to pay attention to experience. Gadamer (1975) noted that:

'The opening up and keeping open of possibilities is only possible because we find ourselves deeply interested in that which makes the question possible in the first place. To truly question something is to interrogate something from the heart of our existence, from the centre of our being.' (p. 266)

If things do not matter then they are not cared for and neglected. When those things are people then the significance of the practitioner's commitment becomes self-evident. Commitment balances or harmonises conflict to convert and mobilise life-consuming or negative energy into life-enhancing or positive energy to fuel the necessary action to resolve contradiction. We pay attention to our experience even when issues are painful. Rogers (1969) believed that a small child is ambivalent about learning to walk; he stumbles, he falls, he hurts himself. It is a painful process. Yet, the satisfaction of developing his potential far outweighs the bumps and bruises. Nurses often reflect on painful situations. Without doubt, many practitioners will lack the commitment necessary for reflection because looking at self and self's practice is too painful. Practice is not always a pretty sight and practitioners may be motivated to avoid the self gaze. I have worked with many practitioners who lack a strong sense of commitment about their practice. Such loss of commitment is always evident across their pattern of being and is a trigger for discussion within guided reflection – 'I can sense you don't want to be here today'.

Yet the realisation of caring as a consequence of learning through the painful experience is profoundly satisfying. Satisfaction is positive feedback to nourish commitment and reaffirm beliefs. To cite Van Manen (1990):

'Retrieving or recalling the essence of caring is not a simple matter of simple etymological analysis or explication of the usage of the word. Rather, it is the construction of a way of life to live the language of our lives more deeply, to become more truly who we are when we refer to ourselves [as nurses].' (p. 59)

Karen noted the flowering of her commitment to her practice and reflection:

'Sessions 1–6 were very much led by the supervisor, but in session 7 we had a sudden breakthrough and I took control. From then on I felt I was growing through supervision – I remember telling Chris I felt like a seedling in spring which has felt the sun and is now growing big and strong into a tree.'

The growth of commitment to herself and consequently to her practice was an emotional experience for Karen. She noted how she increasingly looked forward to her sessions: 'I knew how much I benefited, but I also knew how much energy it took and I often felt drained afterwards'. (Johns, 1998a, p. 225).

Initially Karen had felt ambivalent at the perceived threat of having her level of competence exposed and the recognition that her previous ways of coping were no longer congruent with desirable practice. As practitioners become more reflective they become increasingly committed to practice because they receive constant positive feedback about the value of themselves and the impact of their caring practice on patients' lives. Practitioners come to feel valued within a positive reinforcing spiral.

Contradiction

Contradiction, between what is desirable and actual practice as known through reflection, is the fundamental learning opportunity of reflection. As such, the practitioner needs to know and focus what is desirable and reflect in ways whereby actual practice is not distorted.

Conflict

Contradiction is felt as conflict. Conflict is *the* driving force for learning through reflection. The stronger the felt conflict within contradiction, the more likely the person will take action as a consequence (Kieffer, 1984). The stronger the practitioner's commitment about her practice, then the stronger the felt sense of contradiction when reflection indicates to her that her beliefs have been contradicted within her practice. Empowerment theory indicates that people take action because of felt conflict and strongly held beliefs (Kieffer, 1984).

Challenge

The natural tendency may be to protect self from conflict, leading the practitioner to rationalise the felt contradiction and weaken the force of conflict. As such it may be difficult for the practitioner to reflect effectively without the balanced challenge and support of a guide. Balance is significant in avoiding either threat – too much challenge – or comfort – too little challenge (see p. 59).

Catharsis

The trigger for reflection is often some strong emotion or residual feeling (Boyd & Fales, 1983). When practitioners struggle to know what to write in a reflective journal, I suggest commencing with the feeling 'I feel sad, guilty, angry, frustrated, joyful', etc. Catharsis enables the practitioner to express these feelings (Heron, 1975). Only then can the practitioner begin to explore the source of the feeling and understand why she felt as she did (Boud *et al.*, 1985). Releasing the energy tied up in negative feelings for positive action is a significant source of energy for reflection.

Creation

Within any reflection on experience, the practitioner considers how she has responded within the particular situation and challenges herself to identify and explore other, more effective ways in which she might have responded and considers the consequences. In this way, she is constantly expanding her ability to interpret or frame situations in action and develop her repertoire of appropriate responses.

Reflection is always anticipating the future, planting new seeds of insights and ways of responding that can intuitively or deliberately be drawn upon in new situations.

Connection

Reflection enables the practitioner to connect new insights on different levels.

- With self – 'who am I?'. This connection takes place on one level within practice itself and on another level by reflecting on experience.
- Self with the experience of others – 'who am I?' in context of 'who others are', both patients and colleagues within the particular situation.
- The present experience with past experiences whilst anticipating future practice (see Temporal framing, p. 65).
- Ideal options for action with the real world of practice (see Reality perspective framing, p. 65).

Caring

The outcome of reflection is more desirable and effective practice or, in other words, realising the caring self in terms of the impact of self within practice. When reflection on experience is guided, the relationship between guide and practitioner mirrors the caring relationship between practitioner and patient. Both occupy therapeutic spaces to enable the patient or practitioner to learn through experience even though the context of what is deemed therapeutic is very different.

Congruence

Reflection is a holistic approach to development congruent with a holistic approach to health care. It commences with the person's experience and enables the person to find meaning in the particular situation with the intention of gaining insight, making the best decisions and taking appropriate action. The greater the congruence between caring in practice and developmental processes, the greater the learning potential and the less risk of creating contradiction.

Constructing knowing

Reflection is a doorway to access personal knowing that has generally been thought of as difficult to articulate. Schön (1983) noted that:

> 'When we go about the spontaneous intuitive performance of the actions of everyday life, we show ourselves to be knowledgeable in some way. Often we cannot say what it is that we know. When we try to describe it we find ourselves at a loss, or we produce descriptions that are obviously inappropriate. Our knowing is ordinarily tacit, implicit in our patterns of action and in our feel for the stuff with which we are dealing. It seems right to say that our knowing is in our doing.' (p. 49)

By telling stories and using structured reflection, tacit patterns of action and intuitive performance are examined, leading to greater understanding of the way the self responds within situations. New insights and ideas are constantly applied to future situations and subsequently reflected on, leading to a spiral of reflexive knowing. Within this process the practitioner draws on relevant extant theory to inform practice which then becomes assimilated into personal knowing.

Growth of 'voice'

The construction of personal knowing can be viewed as the growth of 'voice', a metaphor for empowerment (Belenky *et al.*, 1986) to describe the way people develop an informed and assertive voice through a series of levels (Box 3.3).

Box 3.3   Developmental stages of 'finding voice' (Belenky *et al.*, 1986).

Silence
Received knowledge
Subjective knowledge: the inner voice – the quest for self
Procedural knowledge
- Separate knowing
- Connected knowing
Constructed knowledge

Silence

At the level of silence, many practitioners may feel intimidated about speaking out and challenging more powerful others who limit their ability to articulate and assert their point of view. Writing and sharing stories gives the nurse a voice.

Received knowledge

At the level of received knowledge, practitioners speak only through the words of others. 'We do it this way because we are told to.' From this perspective practitioners are empty vessels too full with instruction to do things in approved ways, always dependent on others. Received knowledge comprises a non-questioning conformity, lack of initiative, lack of responsibility, inflexible decision making and routine practice.

Subjective knowing

At the level of subjective knowing, the practitioner's opinions are clearly heard and valued by self, yet they may be relatively uninformed and hence lack authority. It is at this level that the practitioner's knowing is grounded in experience and relationships with others. Belenky *et al.* (1986) note:

> 'During the period of subjective knowing, women lay down procedures for systematically learning and analysing experience. But what seems distinctive in these women is that their strategies for knowing grow out of their very embeddedness in human relationships and their alertness to the details of everyday life. Subjectivist women value what they see and hear around them and begin to feel a need to understand the people with whom they live and who impinge on their lives. Though they may be emotionally or intellectually isolated from others at this point in their histories, they begin to actively analyse their past and current interactions with others.' (p. 85)

At this level, practitioners accept ownership of their experience. Writing and sharing stories with others begins a process of connection with others. They come out of isolation. The quest for self is a restlessness to fulfil self. It is this spark that is nurtured and fanned through reflection.

Procedural knowledge

At the level of procedural knowledge, the practitioner begins to speak with a more informed voice. The *connected knower* is informed by empathic experience through tuning into the experience of the other within the existential dialogue. The *separate knower* is informed through a critical appreciation of theory. Nothing is taken at face value but examined for its meaning yet in a detached, objective manner very distinct from the connected knower.

Constructed knowledge

At the level of constructed knowledge the practitioner weaves together the subjective and procedural voices to speak with an informed, passionate and assertive voice. The work within guided reflection is explicitly aimed at the development of the constructed voice by integrating the subjective and procedural voices (Johns & Hardy, 1998).

Significance of intuition

To re-visit the words that commenced Schön's quote (p. 40): 'When we go about the spontaneous intuitive performance . . .' Schön's work, in discussing the knowledge that professionals need to practise, highlighted the way that practitioners work in the messy, swampy lowlands where there are few answers to the unfolding drama of everyday practice. Perhaps this is nowhere more true than in nursing, where nurses daily confront situations of distress and conflict within the unfolding human encounter. Having no prescription at hand, practitioners draw on previous experience and intuition to them how to proceed. As such, the practitioner's voice is largely in reflecting her deeply embodied sense of personal knowing in practic type of intuitive knowing is subjective, contextualised and transcended through new experiences.

Benner (1984), drawing on the model of skill acquisition (Dreyfus & Dreyfus, 1986), researched the development of expertise, drawing a continuum from novice to expert. The model of skill acquisition holds that experts tend to respond to situations intuitively. If this is true, and there is no reason to doubt it, then reflection offers a tangible way to develop intuition by increasing sensitivity within situations. Knowing in practice stands in sharp contrast to a view of nursing knowledge as being 'objective', decontextualised and claiming universal application in the form of theory. This latter form of knowledge has been claimed as necessary for nursing's disciplinary knowledge base because it can be observed and verified (Kikuchi, 1992). Historically, professions such as nursing have accepted the superiority of technical knowledge over more subjective forms of knowing (Schön, 1983). As Visinstainer (1986) noted:

> 'Even when nurses govern their own practice, they succumb to the belief that the "soft stuff" such as feelings and beliefs and support are not quite as substantive as the hard data from laboratory reports and sophisticated monitoring.' (p. 37)

The consequence of this position in nursing has been the repression of other forms of knowledge which has perpetuated the oppression of nurses and of their clinical nursing knowledge (Street, 1992). Since the Briggs Report (DHSS, 1972) emphasised that nursing should be a research-based profession, nursing has endeavoured to respond to this challenge. However, the general understanding of what 'research based' means has followed a positivist pathway reflecting a dominant agenda to explain and predict events. Researchers who have endeavoured to understand why research is not used in practice (Hunt, 1981; Armitage, 1990) have suggested that the blame lies with the practitioners for their failure to access and utilise research. Schön (1983) has argued that little research has been done to address the real problems of everyday practice and that research always needs to be interpreted for its significance within the particular situation. The decontextualised nature of most research makes this a difficult if not impossible task. Schön exposes an illusion that research has answers that can simply be applied.

Cioffi (1997), drawing on the work of Tversky & Kahneman (1973, 1974), suggests that judgements made in uncertain conditions are most commonly heuristic in nature. Such processes are servants to intuition. The heuristics intend to improve the probability of getting intuition right by linking the current intuition to past experience, being able to see the salient points within any situation and having a baseline position to judge against. Without doubt, the majority of decisions are intuitive within the moment rather than deliberative processes. King & Appleton (1997) and Cioffi (1997) endorse the significance of intuition within decision making and action following their review of the research literature and rhetoric on intuition; reflection accesses, values and develops intuitive processes (Cioffi, 1997). The practitioner's intuitive response to a situation is a non-deliberative yet considered response that draws on the practitioner's tacit knowing in order to respond adequately. In this context, tacit means embodied yet not conscious ways of knowing based on a perception of the whole situation.

Writing a reflective journal

Tony's story was written in my reflective journal. Reflection on experience focuses attention on a meaningful event. Writing reflections in a journal creates a space in often busy and distracted lives to focus on self, to look in at self and acknowledge who we are. This is important work for people such as nurses who use the self as a therapeutic tool. The need to know and manage self is vital if we are to be available to the other person. Hall (1964) noted that the nurse, in order to use herself therapeutically, must know 'who she is so that her own concerns will not interfere with the patient's exploration of his concerns' (p. 152).

Imagine clinical practice as a fast-moving river. In the busyness of the day, many practitioners feel they are being swept along in the current, reacting to events as they unfold about them. Imagine an eddy within the fast-moving water that enables the practitioner to swim out of the current in order to reflect on events. The eddy is still part of the dynamic harmony of events, it is not time out from the river itself. Yet the current is strong and the effort to find the eddy requires vision and resolve. Initiatives such as clinical supervision now provide a legitimate opportunity for reflection.

Yet can guided reflection become a meaningful and practical endeavour to connect the practitioner's beliefs about practice with the realities of everyday whitewater rafting across the furious river of practice? Some practitioners relish the excitement and challenge of whitewater rafting, others cling on for grim death. It is always tiring and dangerous despite the apparent safety precautions. My journal, like an eddy, is a quiet place. It is a place where I can gather my scattered thoughts. Rinpoche (1992), in talking about the need for meditation, says:

> 'We are fragmented into so many different aspects. We don't know who we really are, or what aspects of ourselves we should identify with or believe in. So many contradictory voices, dictates, and feelings fight for control over our inner lives that we find ourselves scattered everywhere, in all directions, leaving nobody at home. Meditation [reflection] then helps to bring the mind home.' (p. 59)

Reflection is a place to listen and pay attention to one's own heartbeat of experience. How often do we listen to what our heart tells us?

Through reflection, the practitioner comes to know 'who I am' and to make 'who I am' increasingly available for therapeutic work. As George Elliot wrote in *Daniel Deronda* 'There is a great deal of unmapped country within us which would have to be taken into account in an explanation of our gusts and storms. Reflection is mapping, charting the unknown area, expanding the Johari window to reveal self to self and others (Box 3.4).

Box 3.4   Johari window (Luft, 1970).

	Behaviour known to self	Behaviour unknown to self
Behaviour known to others	**Public**	**Blind**
Behaviour unknown to others	**Hidden**	**Unknown**

In his book *Awakenings*, Sacks (1976) says:

> 'In the study of our most complex sufferings and disorder of being we are compelled to scrutinise the deepest, darkest, and most fearful parts of ourselves, the parts we all strive to deny or not to see. The thoughts which are most difficult to grasp or express are those which awaken in us our strongest denials and our most profound intuitions.' (p. 15)

As an experienced reflective journalist I do not follow any technique in writing my journal although such techniques are available to guide practitioners (see below). My writing is a process of unfolding significance and meaning, usually triggered by some strong emotion, often a sense of unease about some aspect of that day's practice – the C for catharsis. I reflect on my anxiety, emotion, concern, joy, anger, frustration. Reflection helps me to view these emotions and put them into perspective. In the process of writing I pay attention to these feelings that might otherwise be suppressed or rationalised. Reflection gives me the opportunity to accept and explore the emotion, to understand it and to learn from it. In working through the feeling or thought, I can transcend it and use the negative energy in positive ways to contemplate future actions. Blackwolf Jones & Jones (1996) illuminate what this process may feel like.

> 'What dark caves must you walk through? What do you fear? What are the things that make you swallow hard or tighten your jaw? What memories still bite you? What situations or people do you avoid, postpone, run away from or aggressively

blast through? These are your dark caves. Take the time to write these things down. Become intimate with your fears, for if you pretend they don't exist they are empowered, and then, they rule your life. Learn to walk through your fear. It is okay to be afraid and nervous and scared. You will not break. Each time you walk through your fear you become stronger and fear becomes weaker. Each time you walk through your fear you learn more about yourself. What possibilities await you? Knowing the colours of your strengths, fears, challenges and joy, what possibilities appear? Your dance can be danced with a variety of steps, a variety of expressions, a variety of emotion. Keep a journal of your strengths, fears, challenges and possibilities. Add to it when you can, Reflect on this often. Take the time to look over the results of the above discoveries. This is a mirror of your Self. From this reflection, the final dance will appear.' (p. 52–3)

Accessing reflection

Read Tony's story again and consider the pattern of the reflective account. Recognising a pattern suggests that a *technique* may be useful, at least initially, in guiding the practitioner to reflect. In my experience of guiding reflection, many practitioners struggle to know how to reflect. Whilst many reflective structures are available within the literature, I have developed the model for structured reflection (MSR) as a technique to guide the practitioner's reflection (Box 3.5). The MSR was constructed through analysing the pattern of dialogue between the practitioner and guide within guided reflection relationships and framed with Strauss & Corbin's grounded theory paradigm model (Johns, 1998c). The MSR has been reflexively developed through reflection on its use in practice, resulting in the 12th edition.

Looking in

Rinpoche (1992) says 'Our minds have two positions: looking out and looking in'. Rinpoche is essentially talking about meditation, yet reflection can be likened to meditation in many ways. Rinpoche again:

'I think we do, sometimes, half understand glimpses of the nature of mind, experienced as a moment of illumination, peace, bliss, but modern culture gives us no context or framework in which to comprehend them. Worse still, rather than encouraging us to explore these glimpses more deeply and discover where they spring from, we are told in both obvious and subtle ways to shut them out. We know that no one will take us seriously if we try to share them. So we ignore what could really be the most revealing experiences of our lives, if only we understood them. This is perhaps the darkest and most disturbing aspect of modern civilisation – its ignorance and repression of who we really are.' (p. 50–51)

Looking in encourages the practitioner to pause amidst the hectic pace of life and find quiet space to focus on thoughts and feelings that arise in

Box 3.5 Model for structured reflection.

Looking in
- Find a space to focus on self.
- Pay attention to your thoughts and emotions.
- Write down those thoughts and emotions that seem significant in realising desirable work.

Looking out
- Write a description of the situation surrounding your thoughts and feelings.
- What issues seem significant?
- Aesthetics
    What was I trying to achieve?
    Why did I respond as I did?
    What were the consequences of that for the patient/others/myself?
    How were others feeling?
    How did I know this?
- Personal
    Why did I feel the way I did within this situation?
- Ethics
    Did I act for the best? (ethical mapping)
- What factors (either embodied within me or embedded within the environment) were influencing me?
- Empirics
    What knowledge did or could have informed me?
- Reflexivity
    Does this situation connect with previous experiences?
    How could I handle this situation better?
    What would be the consequences of alternative actions for the patient/others/myself?
    How do I *now* feel about this experience?
    Can I support myself and others better as a consequence?
    How 'available' am I to work with patients/families and staff to help them meet their needs?

consciousness. A great benefit of clinical supervision is this opportunity to take time out to reflect with another person. I currently guide a ward sister who works with patients experiencing disfiguring cancer. In our first two sessions she shared two stories concerning her sense of guilt that she had not been as caring as she might have been. She had gone home dissatisfied. She suffered. Yet she is the most caring of people. It was painful to look in at herself. Her natural inclination was to judge herself harshly. Why is that? Why do we give ourselves such a hard time? Perhaps she, like you, has internalised an idealised state of being a nurse that can never be attained. She certainly embodied the idea that good nurses cope and if we struggle in the face of another's suffering, we are somehow inadequate. Perhaps it is no wonder we always view ourselves so negatively and why we might naturally avoid reflection. In the third session she shared two experiences of great joy

that illustrated the ways in which she had connected with two sets of relatives, easing their distress. In just three sessions she had come to look at
herself differently. Rinpoche (1992) again:

> 'Let's say we turn away from looking in one direction. We have been taught to
> spend our lives chasing our thoughts and projections. We are so addicted to
> looking outside ourselves that we have lost access to our inner being almost
> completely. We are terrified to look inward, because our culture has given us no
> idea of what we will find. So we make our lives so hectic that we eliminate the
> slightest risk of looking into ourselves... In a world dedicated to distraction,
> silence and stillness terrify us; we protect ourselves from them with noise and
> frantic busyness. (p. 51–2)... So, have a spacious, open and compassionate atti-
> tude towards your thoughts and emotions. When we do not intrinsically under-
> stand what they are then our thoughts become the seeds of confusion. Before them
> "be like a wise old man, watching a child play".' (p. 74)

In order to cope or maintain a facade of coping, practitioners close
themselves to themselves yet in doing so, they close themselves to others.
They become unable to care on a deep level of connection necessary for
holistic practice. In denying themselves, they deny the possibility of realising
self as caring.

Looking out

Like the Burford NDU model, the MSR offers a series of reflective cues that
focus the practitioner's attention on significant issues within experience. One
practitioner wrote:

> 'I personally feel that I would have been lost without the model for structured
> reflection that I used for my journal keeping. I fear this would have remained at the
> descriptive level. Describing events but not knowing what to do with the descrip-
> tions is almost like sitting in a car without wheels, forever stuck on the starting line
> of reflection without the ability to move down the road to being a more effective
> practitioner.' [Graham cited in Johns, 1997a, p. 91–2)

The MSR cues are arranged in a logical order, enabling a progression of
thought. I have utilised the work of Carper (1978) to tune the cues into
discrete areas of knowledge (this work is discussed on pp. 77–8) although
this has only educational rather than practical value.

Many models of reflection are set out as reflective cycles – for example,
Gibbs (1988; see Box 3.6). Indeed, Bond & Holland (1998) have converted
the MSR into a cyclical process. This might be useful for the novice reflective
practitioner but remember, within a reflective perspective such structures as
the MSR are merely devices to help you reflect rather than impose a prescription of what reflection is. However, practitioners do not reflect in neat

Box 3.6 The reflective cycle (Gibbs, 1988).

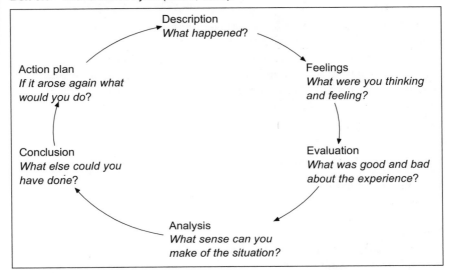

stages. It appears to be a much more holistic process. In a technological society the risk exists that the MSR will be grasped as a technology and used in concrete ways. This is evident in models of nursing that constantly fit the patient into the model's schema. The result is to obscure rather than clarify 'who a person is'. From a technological perspective, the risk is that the practitioner will strive to fit her experience to the model rather than use the model creatively to see herself in context of the particular experience. Rinpoche (1992) believes that:

> 'Largely because of our Western technological culture people tend to be absorbed by what I would call "the technology of meditation" [reflection]. The modern world, after all, is fascinated by mechanisms and machines, and addicted to purely practical formulae. But by far the most important feature of meditation [reflection] is not the technique, but the spirit: the skilful, inspired, and creative way in which we practise, which could also be called "the posture".' (p. 64–5)

Posture is the location of quiet time, letting feelings and thoughts come to mind and writing about the situation around such thoughts. Only then can a more cognitive *looking out* help to challenge self within the situation, gain insights, identify and contemplate new ways of responding in similar situations. Holly (1989) noted:

> 'It [keeping a journal] makes possible new ways of theorizing, reflecting on and coming to know one's self. Capturing certain words while the action is fresh, the author is often provoked to question why ... writing taps tacit knowledge; it brings into awareness that which we sense but could not explain.' (p. 71–5)

Reflective media

In challenging the idea of reflection as a cognitive activity, reflection may be triggered by more 'right brain' activity – for example, using painting, poetry, sculpturing and dance to express thoughts and feelings around specific experience. Right brain activity is associated with creativity and sensitivity, essential attributes of caring practice. I use a number of poems in this book to express my own ideas. Leslie shared a poem with me in one guided session to reflect his feelings about a patient's death.

Remembering MA – a patient

Walking on a high wire above the trees.
Below me is a broad river,
over-ripe with death.
From holding death's hand,
Looking death in the eye.
washing and dressing death,
Laying death out
and wrapping death in a sheet, yet
There is no understanding.

Dry, flaking skin stretched over bones
sticking together in a creaking frame,
so frail – it seems crushable.
Holding hands with life,
feeling life fade
away with last labour gasps –
death creeps in.

I have heard the scream of love
and gathered the tears.
This bundle of dead cells
is not the one we knew
who once cried in her mother's arms,
walked her first step.
Whose laugh and early words
lit her parents' eyes.
This bundle of dead cells is not the lover once
caressed and hugged close, nor
yet a wife, a mother, a friend
– she has gone
and lives in the mind only, and
caught in photographs.

Her friend told the nurse:
'Nobody else understood her.
Nobody else knew her like I did.'
There is no understanding.

'Leslie'

Guided reflection as a developmental process

Caring in practice is made manifest, known & developed through guided reflection.

Reflection on experience, either alone in a reflective journal or guided by another, is the fourth caring dialogue which enables the practitioner to develop and synchronise the other caring dialogues (see Box 2.6).

Reflective writing is a constant creative process of interpretation. It requires an openness, authenticity and commitment to self as caring. However, there are limits to reflecting alone. Practitioners often refer with emotional intensity to the importance of the external enabler (Kieffer, 1984). Perhaps this emotional intensity is related to the fact that practitioners bring situations of emotional disturbance, grounded in such feelings as guilt, anger, distress, anxiety and conflict, to guided reflection. The practitioner presents in crisis. The guide or supervisor works with the practitioner to help them find meaning in the event, in order to understand and learn through it and to emerge at a higher level of consciousness (Newman 1994). The constant process of checking out the adequacy of interpretation counters any criticism that the stories are mere anecdotes riddled with unsupported assumptions.

The need for guidance

Tony's story illustrated the potential of reflection as a meaningful way for the practitioner to connect with her deeper self, to know herself in authentic ways. Perhaps nurses, through their formative experiences, have lost connection with their deeper selves in the face of a health-care culture that does not seem to value caring and yet confronts the nurse with daily events of suffering and deep distress. When this work is not acknowledged and valued, then nurses may need to find ways of coping that desensitise the nurse to herself. This is particularly apposite within a culture where a good nurse is expected to cope. Jourard (1971) considered that this inevitably leads to self-alienation. Because nurses have learnt to protect themselves at a deep level, they may need guidance to help them face themselves and learn to cope in non-desensitising ways. The practitioner may also need guidance because of the difficulty in viewing practice from different perspectives. Using a window as a metaphor, O'Donohue (1997) says:

'Many people remain trapped at the one window, looking out every day at the same scene in the same way. Real growth is experienced when you draw back from that one window, turn and walk around the inner tower of the soul and see all the different windows that await your gaze. Through these different windows, you can see new vistas of possibility, presence and creativity. Complacency, habit and blindness often prevent you from feeling your life. So much depends on the frame of vision – the window through which we look.' (p. 163–4]

The need to guide reflection can be summarised as follows.

- To expose contradiction and emphasise felt conflict.

- To expose and confront self-distortion and limited horizons and to challenge the practitioner to look at situations from new perspectives. Cox *et al.* (1991) focus this phenomenon:

  'Reflection in isolation is difficult to sustain because of the difficulty in surfacing and transcending what may be our own distorted self understandings, asking ourselves difficult, often self-exposing questions, facing the difficult answers to such questions, and, perhaps most particularly, keeping our vision directed towards new possibilities for understanding and action.' (p. 385)

- To unearth and understand the factors that have limited the ability to achieve desirable and effective work.

- To nurture a commitment that may have become numbed or blunted when working in 'unsympathetic' environments. In nurturing commitment, the supervisor accepts the practitioner whatever her position. If the practitioner is numbed towards her practice, then this is the point of connection. The practitioner may be wounded and defensive. As such, the supervisor reads the signs and shines a gentle light to help the practitioner to see and know who she is. In an outcome-oriented health-care culture, the temptation may be to shine a bright aggressive light that frightens the practitioner caught in the glare.

- To gain new insights and discover and explore new ways of responding within situations.

- To penetrate critical levels of reflection that may be outside the scope of the practitioner reflecting by herself. Consider the question 'Is reflection a natural phenomenon?'. Perhaps all people reflect to some extent as a natural response to situations that provoke anxiety. Using the levels of reflective consciousness set out by Mezirow (1981), Powell (1989), in a small study with eight nurses, indicated that they did not naturally reflect at a critical consciousness level. Mezirow identified six levels of reflective consciousness; moving from consciousness, to critical consciousness (Box 3.7), suggesting that reflection can be perceived in terms of depth. Van

Box 3.7   Mezirow's levels or reflectivity.

Consciousness

Affective reflectivity – becoming aware of how we feel about things
Discriminant reflectivity – perceiving the relationships between things
Judgemental reflectivity – becoming aware of how we make value judgements

Critical consciousness

Conceptual reflectivity – questioning the adequacy and morality of concepts
Psychic reflectivity – recognising one's own prejudices and the impact of these on judgement and action
Theoretical reflectivity – understanding self in the context of desirable action

---

Manen (1977) identified three levels of functional reflection. The first level was asking 'how questions', concerned with technique. The second level was 'why questions', concerned with reason. The third level was concerned with examining the conditions of practice, 'why do things exist as they do and how do they need to change in order to enable effective practice?'. It is at this level that the taken for granted is made problematic. Van Manen considered that, generally, people did not reflect on this level.

- To support practitioners to become empowered to take appropriate action to resolve contradiction. Lieberman (1989; cited by Day, 1993) commented: 'working in bureaucratic settings has taught everyone to be compliant, to be rule governed, not to ask questions, seek alternatives or deal with competing values.' (p. 88). In response, Day (1993) asserts that reflection will bring the practitioner into tension with prevailing dominant organisational values, suggesting that reflection will struggle to make an impact unless the organisation is sympathetic to the collaborative philosophy of reflection.

> 'Success will depend in part on the culture of the organization. Where the unspoken values underlying reflective practice clash with prevailing [school] culture, tensions will arise. Traditional leadership and followship roles must move towards partnerships which embody collegial rather than adversarial relationships, and in which power is equalised.' (p. 88)

Picking up the last point, it is difficult to envisage such cultural shifts. The participants in Kieffer's (1984) study of empowerment referred with great emotional intensity to the importance of the external enabler to support the practitioner's struggle against more powerful others who are motivated to maintain the status quo. The practitioner connects with her guide as a representative of the wider community, the gatekeeper and guide to this world. In order to do this, the guide must connect with the practitioner in terms of her existing reality and, simultaneously, in terms of a potential new reality. Fay (1987) noted that:

'Coming to a radically new self-conception is hardly ever a process that occurs simply by reading some theoretical work; rather it requires an environment of trust and support in which one's own preconceptions and feeling can be properly made conscious to oneself, in which one can think through one's experiences in terms of a radically new vocabulary which expresses a fundamentally different conceptualisation of the world in which one can see the particular and concrete ways that one unwittingly collaborates in producing one's own misery and in which one can gain emotional strength to accept and act on one's new insights.' (p. 265–6)

The guide is a powerful person and the attitudes and expertise she brings to the relationship are obviously critical to the developmental process. Who the guide should be is a critical issue that is explored later in this chapter. It is essential that the guide is a reflective practitioner able to:

- facilitate the practitioner to reflect in purposeful ways
- learn through her own experience of guiding the practitioner
- remain available to the practitioner within the unfolding moment

Humanistic learning

A number of points of congruence between guided reflection and humanistic learning can be stated.

- Reflection enables practitioners to pay attention to those things that matter to them. This is highlighted in adult learning theory (Knowles, 1980), which recognises that adults are ready to learn material relevant to their life situation.
- The supervisor and practitioner actively work towards creating a milieu of trust whereby the practitioner feels safe to disclose experiences. The supervisor critically manages her own prejudices and power and recognises and values the practitioner's viewpoints.
- The practitioner's real world of practice is the learning milieu in which new insights and new ways of acting can be applied and tested through future actions.
- Learning is facilitated when the student participates responsibly in the learning process. Rogers (1969) noted:

  'When he chooses his own directions, helps to discover his own learning resources, formulates his own problems, decides his own course of action, lives with the consequences of these choices, then significant learning is maximised.'

Hence, an explicit aim of guided reflection is to enable the practitioner to accept responsibility for self-development.

- Learning through guided reflection engages the whole of the practitioner within the learning experience. Rogers noted:

  'Self-initiated learning which involves the whole person of the learner – feelings as well as intellect – is the most lasting and pervasive.'

- Practitioners tend to pay attention to experience because of strong emotional aspects.
- The reflective practitioner embodies reflection as a natural process, enabling each unfolding experience to become a learning opportunity.

The therapeutic milieu of guided reflection

Creating a therapeutic relationship between the supervisor and practitioner is fundamental to guided reflection, mirroring the therapeutic relationship between nurse and patient. In creating the therapeutic relationship, at least five factors are significant:

(1) Contracting
(2) Creating a climate for practitioner disclosure
(3) Balancing challenge with support
(4) Constructing meaning
(5) Framing perspectives

Contracting

'If supervision is to become and remain a co-operative experience which allows for real rather than token accountability, a clear, even tough, working agreement needs to be negotiated. The agreement needs to provide sufficient safety and clarity for the student/worker to know where she stands; and it needs sufficient teeth for the supervisor to feel free and responsible for making the challenges...' (Hawkins & Shohet, 1989, p. 29)

I assume the practitioner has a choice of guide and also a choice of whether or not to enter guided reflection. As such, the contracting process is concerned with the practitioner and guide deciding whether to work with each other. This involves discussing mutual backgrounds and expectations, the processes of learning and monitoring development and pragmatics such as how frequently to meet.

One key expectation is that the practitioner will accept responsibility for what takes place within guided reflection. However, the practitioner may not know what to expect or how to respond within guided reflection. Therefore, the guide nurtures the practitioner's empowerment to accept responsibility for the supervision relationship and in doing so, to accept responsibility for ensuring and monitoring her own practice.

Who should the guide be?

The practitioner's relationship with the guide is critical to the success of guided reflection. One contemporary debate fostered by the advent of clinical supervision is whether the guide (or clincial supervisor) should be the line manager or somebody in a non-line management relationship either within or external to the organisation. I have been both a line manager guide and non-line manager guide. Box 3.8 sets out the relative advantages and disadvantages. The advantages are very powerful, equated with enabling the line manager supervisor to fulfil any clinical leadership role. My own experience of implementing guided reflection at Burford was very significant as it offered me a collaborative way of working with primary and associate nurses to facilitate their development of clinical effectiveness and role fulfilment. Creating collaborative relationships is considered necessary for primary nursing (Manthey, 1980). As a consequence, our ways of relating within guided reflection spilled out to become new ways of relating within practice itself. From this perspective, the development potential for the guide/manager is evident.

Box 3.8   The potential advantages and disadvantages of line management guidance (Johns and McCormack, 1998).

Advantages of line manager guide/ supervisor	Disadvantages of line manager guide/ supervisor
• Understands the practitioner's practice • Can tackle situations together • Work towards a 'new type' of relationship based on openness and authenticity • Spillover of supervision work into everyday practice • Mutual growth and empowerment • Work together to realise a shared vision of practice • Opportunity to acknowledge and value practitioners	• Need to 'fix it' • Paternalistic – takes action of behalf of the practitioner • Supervises as she manages, reinforcing dependency and hierarchical norms • Conflict over what's best – threat to hierarchical control • Manipulates agenda to suit own needs • Supervision seen as moulding an ideal practitioner or being remedial • Takes on board practitioner's distress • 'Maternal role for hurt child' – cannot detach self from situation • Lack of vision in seeing other ways of doing things (tarred with the same brush as the practitioner) • Practitioner may avoid sharing certain types of experiences, especially if grounded in interpersonal conflict with the manager/supervisor

Disadvantages of line management supervision

The disadvantages are more concerned with attitude and technique rather than role.

Perhaps the most significant of these disadvantages are the supervisor's lack of vision beyond 'normal practice' and the constraint of previous learnt hierarchical ways of responding within managerial relationships *despite* collegial intent (Johns & McCormack, 1998). The risk is that the manager/ supervisor wears two hats which do not easily fit together, using the guided reflection space to address her own agenda.

Without doubt, there is a tension between guided reflection or clinical supervision as an emancipatory process enabling practitioners to fulfil their therapeutic destiny and its use as a new technology of surveillance (Johns, 1996a; Johns & McCormack, 1998). Supervisors concerned with their own agendas may abuse supervision by using it as an opportunity to 'correct' faulty practitioners, especially from a line management bureaucratic perspective. The risk is that guided reflection or supervision becomes a managerial tool rather than an emancipatory process grounded in the practitioner's agenda. If so, the practitioner is likely to resist or comply with expectations and the potential developmental opportunity will be diminished.

Consider who might guide your reflection. What factors influenced your choice?

Creating a climate for practitioner disclosure

The *sine qua non* of guided reflection is creating a therapeutic space in which the practitioner feels safe to disclose and explore her experiences. Practitioners often feel uncomfortable with this self-scrutiny, as it may lead to the breakdown of facades of competence and reveal ways of coping that are inadequate. Cox (1988) structures this therapeutic space in terms of three dimensions: time, depth and mutuality.

- Time – to judge the pace of events
- Depth – to judge the depth of probing the disclosure
- Mutuality – to judge the involvement and mutual disclosure

On each dimension the issue is *judgement*, which requires the supervisor to read the situation accurately in order to respond appropriately. Mutuality requires a positive regard that the other is a worthy person who can succeed. Otherwise the relationship becomes forced, with a potential for game playing that closes the therapeutic space.

The essence of guided reflection is to establish a reflective dialogue that parallels the existential dialogue between the practitioner and the patient. The supervisor seeks to be available to the practitioner in much the same way as the practitioner seeks to be available to work with the patient or family.

Perhaps the two most significant factors to consider in establishing a safe yet therapeutic space are the supervisor's concern and the management of her own concerns.

Concern is a genuine expression of openness, care, positive regard and authenticity and a willingness to enter into and understand the life of the other from the practitioner's perspective. The following poem, 'River of tears', was my reflection on a very emotional guided reflection session with a ward sister who was very distressed about a situation.

The river of tears

This space between us
A river of tears
Where your tears flow
The flow of pain
Hurt to the quick

This river of tears
Where once your passion flowed
And where passion will flow again
When the clouds have cleared
And the sun can shine again.

And when I gaze across at you
I feel the touch of my concern
My gaze as an eagle's wing
That gently touches the blue
Mood of despair.

The dark woman has broken
I feel her tears flow
Into the dark river that flows between
No words spoken
A clear winter's day within shadow.

I feel the swarms of bees about me
And the song of the bee about me
The dark woman stung
My words to set her free
To move on within this space.

Tears like dewdrops
Sweep across the soft lids
Eyes glisten as the smile breaks through
Her anguished cry stops
In the soft dawn of hope.

Within each tear spilt
I sensed your hopes and fears
Your sense of being betrayed
The machine says tilt
No longer can you play.

Nerve shredded along the edge
This edge your pattern
I sense the ripple
Frailty exposed along the ledge
Step lightly in the dawn.

I am the soul traveller
I meet you within your space
We move beyond . . . co-transcend
The past already just a blur
We have learnt from.

And on another day and in another place
We can look back
And bathe in this river of tears
That flowed within this space
Between our souls.

Christopher Johns

Of course, to equate a supervisor with a soul traveller is poetic licence, although it does highlight the mutuality of supervision, the idea that 'we move beyond'. In working with this ward sister I was very conscious of my therapeutic response to her and subsequently my development of such therapeutic competence. However, concern is a two-edged sword. Even when supervisors are aware of their own concerns it is not necessarily easy to manage these, particularly when the practitioner's actions or attitudes trigger such concerns (Johns, 1998a). Supervisors also need supervision.

The balance of challenge and support

The key learning dynamic within guided reflection is high challenge and high support. Effective guidance is the balance of high challenge to confront contradiction and high support to sustain the commitment, courage and effort to resolve the contradictions and transform self as necessary to become effective in achieving desirable work (Johns, 1996a). Without adequate challenge, the practitioner may rationalise the contradiction and decide not to take appropriate action, particularly where practitioners have been socialised within hierarchical-bureaucratic systems to internalise a sense of the subordinate and powerless self within a coercive management style. As Smyth (1987) notes:

'Most of us, unless we feel uncomfortable, shaken, or forced to look at ourselves, are unlikely to change. It is far easier to accept our current conditions and adopt the least line of resistance.' (p. 40)

Lisa, a Macmillan support nurse in guided reflection with me, noted:

'I felt that being challenged is an essential element of supervision, providing you feel comfortable in your environment and at ease with the supervisor. The challenge element encouraged me to think further than I had been and to deal with issues in a way I would not have considered.' (unpublished supervision notes)

Watering the seeds of doubt

Guidance confronts the practitioner's normal ways of doing things and challenges them to view situations differently. Margolis (1993) considers that new ideas compete with existing ideas. The success of adopting new ideas depends on the robustness of existing ones and the force of argument available to support the new idea. Margolis suggested that habits of mind compete for dominance and thereby generate contradiction. The supervisor's role is to plant seeds of doubt within the landscape of the mind and to water this doubt in order to eventually overthrow the dominant habits of mind that feed an accepted order of things.

Accepting the new idea is just the beginning, the ensuing congruent action cannot be guaranteed. Practitioners do not change simply because they come to understand an issue differently (Fay, 1987; Allen, 1987). This point highlights the folly of imposing liberating structures on people, in that nurses who have been socialised to be powerless are unable to respond to liberating opportunities when they present themselves. The emphasis should be on the practitioners coming to realise a new reality for themselves rather than having this new reality explained to them. For example, all shared experiences concerned with conflict have a fundamental power inequality at their root which manifests itself through different attitudes, beliefs and behaviours. This is not difficult to see or understand provided it is sought and not just taken for granted as part of the 'natural' background of experience. All understanding is cast against the practitioner's background while at the same time the naturalness of social arrangements is challenged so that the practitioner and supervisor can see both the constraints and the potential for change in their situations.

Through the continuity of sessions new ideas can quickly be put into practice and then reflected on as an unfolding experience over time. Guided reflection is a dynamic feedback process that facilitates evolution and growth as practitioners learn through experience to become more effective practitioners. Without guidance, practitioners may reflect in order to rationalise anxiety rather than learn through anxiety. Under these conditions the practitioner may fall back on known ways of responding rather than follow the intuitive lead. Yet even under conditions of anxiety, practitioners' intuitive responses usually hold up. Guidance gives the practitioner positive feedback to reinforce this tacit knowledge and to utilise this 'anxiety' energy in positive ways. Hall (1964) noted:

> 'The energy made available by the body in a state of anxiety can be put to use in exploration of feelings through participation in the struggle to face and solve problems underlying the state of anxiety.' (p. 153)

Constructing meaning

The dialogue between the practitioner and guide/supervisor is a process of co-creating meaning. Dialogue consists of descriptions of experiences and 'connective conversation' – the communication used to facilitate learning, to maintain the flow of supervision and to develop and sustain the supervision relationship. Listening to the practitioner's experience offers the supervisor a number of cues to explore. The process of dialogue unwraps and reconstructs the experience, like peeling back layers of an onion skin to see things for what they are and to explore their significance in terms of the whole.

Open dialogue

Fundamental to an effective collaborative relationship is the creation of the conditions of 'open dialogue', whereby practitioners are free to share their thoughts and feelings without feeling intimidated. Habermas (1984), in his theory of communicative competence, noted the significance within an emancipatory social science of establishing 'ideal speech situations' where people could speak without fear of oppression, the outcome of debate being settled by weight of argument. Open dialogue is necessary for 'co-creating meaning', where the meaning of events is jointly constructed between the supervisor and practitioner. In other words, the supervisor does not impose a meaning on the practitioner from his or her authoritative advantage.

As practitioners learn through experience, their horizons are constantly shifting, as in a developmental process of moving forward. Hence new experience is viewed from a developed position of having learnt through previous experience. When practitioners look back, they can view their journey through the shifting accounts of their reflected experiences. They can see how they have come to talk differently about themselves, reflecting their new understandings and changed actions. Gadamer (1975) highlights how people are always understanding and interpreting themselves in the context of their worlds and the light of their foreknowledge which, from the reflexive viewpoint, is always changing through experience. This looking back and seeing self as a changed person is the essential nature of reflexivity. It is not an endpoint but is always open to and anticipatory of future experiences. Gadamer (1975) noted

'Every experience has implicit horizons before and after, and fuses finally with the continuum of experiences that are present before and after into the unity of the flow of experience.' (cited in Weinsheimer, 1985, p. 157)

Whilst I can help the practitioner recognise her preunderstandings, this is not necessarily reciprocated. My role is to facilitate learning in the other. Issues of clinical knowledge and status also apply despite collegial intent. In other words, the researcher and facilitator may struggle to see how their own prereflective state impacts on the relationship.

'Verbatim' notes are recorded during each session. The notes may not accurately recall what actually happened but they do portray the practitioner's interpretation of that event and hence capture meaning. The issue of accuracy has been raised as a criticism of reflective practice (Newell, 1992) yet it does not matter if the practitioner distorts accuracy because this is done for a reason that can be teased out within the ensuing dialogue. The narratives reveal the vividness of this openness within the developing trust and intimacy of the relationship.

The notes serve a number of purposes.

- To enable the practitioner to agree the content and meaning of the dialogue (*face validity*).
- To enable continuity of dialogue through sessions by picking up issues from the previous session's dialogue.
- To enable the practitioner to reflect further on issues.
- To confront the practitioner with the issues that might otherwise have been denied within the oral mode.
- To provide a record to enable the practitioner to 'look back' and make sense of their experiences/work in guided reflection over time.
- To allow the supervisor to reflect on what was shared within the dialogue and to highlight issues that might be useful to raise in the next session.

Hence the notes bridge the sessions to reinforce the temporal flow of experience over time and capture the nuances of caring.

Framing perspectives

The framing perspectives are a set of lenses used to structure the learning effort through reflection (summarised in Box 3.9). The perspectives were constructed by analysing the pattern of guided reflection dialogue (Johns, 1998a).

Philosophical framing

All practitioners hold beliefs and values about the nature of their nursing practice. I know from holding reflective practice workshops that the over-

Box 3.9 Framing perspectives (Johns, 1997a, 1998a).

- *Philosophical framing* – confronting and clarifying the beliefs/values that constitute desirable practice.
- *Role framing* – clarifying role boundaries/relationships and legitimate authority and power within practice.
- *Theoretical framing* – assimilating theory and research findings with personal knowing.
- *Reality perspective framing* – acknowledging that practising in new ways is not necessarily easy, while helping the practitioner to become knowledgeable and empowered to take necessary action.
- *Temporal framing* – recognising how reflection is not an isolated event but connected through experiences over time in anticipation of future experiences.
- *Problem framing* – focusing problem identification and resolution that emerge through experience.
- *Parallel process framing* – making links between the therapeutic space of guided reflection and clinical practice.
- *Being available* – recognising reflexive learning within the 'being available' template.

whelming majority of practitioners aspire towards holistic practice. Yet what *holistic* means in practice is often not clear. Practitioners also struggle to articulate their beliefs, as if they are buried deep within, perhaps because the contradictions are too obvious or too painful to acknowledge and face. Yet to be effective demands the practitioner's awareness of what being effective means. Where beliefs are inappropriate or contradicted within practice then the practitioner can be guided to confront the meaning and relevance of her beliefs.

Role framing

Role framing challenges the practitioner to clarify her role responsibility and authority to make decisions and take action to fulfil her role responsibility in the context of the particular situation. Issues around role ambiguity and authority are usually in the context of conflict with others where authority for decision making overlaps or blurs.

Primary nurses are directly responsible for the care management of assigned patients, yet responsibility is complex. Box 3.10 sets out the diversity and potentially contradictory nature of the practitioner's responsibility and consequent accountability. Whilst the Burford NDU model espouses a primary responsibility to the patient, it recognises that the traditional culture of health-care organisation and professional dominance asserts the nurse's subordination. The holistic practitioner acknowledges accountability for her actions yet demands respect within interdependent work relationships.

Box 3.10   The diverse nature of practitioner responsibility and accountability.

Accountable to	Rationale
The patient and family	To help them meet their diverse health needs To support the person and family through the medical response
Self	To act with integrity according to beliefs and values and to ensure self-effectiveness
Society	To fulfil and enhance societal expectations of nursing
The organisation	To fulfil role responsibility
The profession	To justify actions within the guidelines of the UKCC Code of Conduct
Peers and co-workers	To work in collaborative and mutually supportive ways to ensure patients and families receive congruent, consistent and effective care

Theoretical framing

The effective practitioner is an informed practitioner who can access and assimilate relevant research findings and theory within her practice. The MSR cue 'what knowledge did or could have informed me?' (see Box 3.5) guides the practitioner to pay attention to theoretical framing. Theory serves to *inform* the reflective practitioner, not to prescribe what she should do or explain what she has done. Brookfield (1987) informs us:

'In trying to find meaning in our lives and to make sense of the things that happen to us, we seek frameworks of understanding that we can impose on the bewildering chaos of our existence.' (p. 45)

Such frameworks need to be viewed through a *sceptical eye* (Dewey, 1933), to ensure that theory is never accepted at face value but examined for its significance. Carper (1978) noted that extant theory always needed to be interpreted creatively within the clinical situation rather than applied as a prescription. Theory is sought and interpreted for its relevance within the specific situation, assimilated and transcended within personal knowing towards constructing what Belenky *et al.* (1986) termed 'constructed knowledge'; the weaving of subjective, connected and separate knowing (see box 3.3). Schön (1987) has stated that the practitioner must always interpret research for its meaning within the context of the particular situation and that theory does not easily fit the complexities of everyday practice situations, which are often indeterminate and defy technical solution. I could not easily have predicted the situations with Tony, even if I had deliberately set out to trigger such conversations.

Supervisors also seem to have difficulty drawing on relevant theory. Brian noted:

'I have not found any common pattern to the way I feed-in theory. On the occasions that I have, it has always felt appropriate and yet I find it difficult to pick out the particular aspects that may be most appropriate. I am conscious of the fine line between theoretical overload and allowing the supervisee to generate their own theory through their reflections.' (Johns, 1998a, p. 271)

Critical dialogue with the literature might be described as a fifth dialogue of caring. The meaningful assimilation of theory into patterns of knowing in practice may only be achieved through reflection.

Reality perspective framing

For many reasons practitioners are unable to take the action they feel they should. Reality perspective framing acknowledges that practitioners live in a real world where forces limit their ability to take action congruent with desired practice. Acknowledgement of this helps to offset any sense of failure. Street (1992) considered such forces to be 'embedded in traditions, historical constructions, and a specific nursing culture. This culture daily shapes nurses and is shaped by them' (p. 254).

Reality framing is a *process-oriented* technique to elicit the reasons why the practitioner could not take the action she felt was appropriate. Failure to acknowledge the practitioner's reality could risk propelling her towards a brick wall of unrealistic expectation that may actually increase her anxiety rather than ease it. Bringing contradiction into consciousness inevitably exposes subconscious ways of defending self, for example rationalisation or projection, that have previously protected the practitioner from the conflict of contradiction. Now these mechanisms become exposed, leaving the practitioner vulnerable (see Chapter 8). Through understanding reality, the masks of self-distortion can be peeled away to reveal the truth whilst supporting ways of focusing on and contemplating new responses.

Temporal framing

Experience is never an isolated event but part of an unfolding temporal narrative that links with past experiences whilst anticipating the future. The practitioner is tuned into this temporal perspective through the reflective cues (MSR; see Box 3.5] 'Does this situation connect with previous situations?' and 'how could I handle this situation better?'.

Temporal framing facilitates the continuity of meaning between present and past experience that Marris (1986) believes is crucial in order to focus on the future in a meaningful way. Each guided reflection builds on the previous session, whereby learning is applied to future experience and subsequently reflected on. This process creates the conditions for reflexivity, looking back and seeing self as a changed person through experience.

So, towards the end of the guided reflection session I ask the practitioner to summarise the session by reflecting on and writing down:

- what has been shared within supervision
- what has been significant in the session
- what actions the practitioner/guide needs to take as a consequence

This helps the practitioner to 'wrap up and package' the session. It also ensures that loose ends are dealt with and the reflective cue 'how do I now feel?' (see Box 3.5) has been addressed. This helps the practitioner to focus her energy to anticipate future practice. When we next meet, the practitioner can reflect on the previous session and the actions she was going to take. Did she take them? What were the consequences? If she didn't take action, then why?

Session by session this record accumulates, providing an account of the practitioner's development which can easily be analysed as a formal review. Reflective review offers the practitioner a formal opportunity to exercise her responsibility for monitoring her own effectiveness (Johns, 1995b). This can be achieved by analysing areas of practice that have been the focus of reflection and making a judgement on whether development has taken place in the light of subsequent situations. Monitoring development may be structured using mapping devices to plot growth, for example managing conflict, becoming assertive, being available, etc. The use of these maps is discussed in subsequent chapters.

Review creates an opportunity to formally integrate guided reflection or clinical supervision within mainstream organisational activity. This can only enhance its value. However, practitioners may have a negative view of appraisal, linking this to some kind of surveillance of performance. Hence, review needs to be contracted at the beginning of guided reflection. The continuity of meaning through experience is enhanced when sessions are held at least every four weeks. Beyond this time span, the sense of continuity weakens significantly, although less so if the practitioner maintains a reflective diary.

Problem framing

The reflective cues within the MSR (Box 3.5) guide the practitioner to pose and clarify problems. It is like framing a picture so its content and borders can be defined and solutions can be envisaged.

Parallel process framing

The relationship between guide and practitioner mirrors the desired therapeutic relationship between practitioner and patient (Box 3.11).

Box 3.11 The parallel between guided reflection and clinical relationship.

Clinical practice relationship	Guided reflection relationship
The practitioner works with the person to help them to find meaning in the experience and make good decisions and take the best action to meet their health needs.	The guide works with the practitioner to help her to find meaning in the experience and make good decisions and take the best action to meet her developmental needs.

Hence, the way the guide responds to the practitioner can be made explicit and considered within the practitioner's experience. For example, consider the dialogue between Helen and her guide (see pp. 178–81) and the way the guide (CJ) uses catharsis and confrontation to help Helen explore her feelings. By making these responses explicit, the guide role models these responses and helps the practitioner consider her own use of these responses within the context of the experience she is reflecting on.

Being available

The being available template offers an empirically constructed framework for the development of becoming an effective practitioner. Within any developmental process it is important to design appropriate ways of monitoring the growth of effective practice. The being available template was constructed by analysing the dialogue between practitioner and guides within guided reflection relationships (Johns, 1997b, 1998a). It is used to structure the account of realising caring in practice in Chapters 4–8.

Chapter 4
Being Available: The Essence of Effective Holistic Practice

Introduction

As a reflective practitioner I nurture my 'knowing self', a self that is sensitive yet critical of self within the caring moment. Through reflection I learn through the experience and transcend previous ways of knowing. My caring is nurtured and renewed as I realise caring as everyday practice.

Being available

In Tony's story, my primary therapeutic effort was to *be available* to help him meet his health needs. The Burford model states 'the extent the nurse can realise caring in practice is determined by the extent she is available to work with the person'. A number of discrete yet interrelated dimensions influence the ability to be available within a holistic perspective.

- Knowing what is desirable
- Knowing the person
- Concern for the person
- The aesthetic response to the person
- Knowing and managing self's involvement with the person
- Creating and sustaining an environment where being available is possible

The 'being available' framework was constructed from an analysis of the experiences practitioners (using the Burford model in everyday practice) shared within guided reflection relationships. The project involved 15 practitioners, sharing over 500 experiences over a four-year continuous research period (Johns, 1998a). Box 4.1 summarises the significance of each dimension.

The extent to which the practitioner knows what desirable means

Knowing what is desirable is reflected in the philosophy of practice. Beliefs and values ripple below the surface of all experience. They motivate and

Box 4.1 The dimensions show the extent to which the practitioner can be available to work with the person in desirable ways.

The extent to which the practitioner knows what 'desirable' means	Knowing what is desirable gives meaning and purpose to practice and focuses concern and action. Within the reflective dialogue, the practitioner's beliefs and values that support desirable practice are exposed and contemplated for their meaning and relevance, enabling contradiction to become evident.
The extent to which the practitioner knows the person	In order to respond appropriately to helping the patient and family, the practitioner needs to know them in the context of the meanings they give to the health event. To achieve this, the practitioner must establish a trusting reflective dialogue with the patient and family where meaning and needs are constantly interpreted within the unfolding moment.
The extent to which the practitioner is concerned for the person	Concern is the motivational expression of caring. Concern creates possibility within the caring relationship (Benner & Wrubel, 1989). The greater the practitioner's concern, the greater the possibilities within her relationship with the patient and family. When the practitioner's concern has become numbed then reasons for this can be explored and understood and concern nurtured to become again a strong passion and motivational force.
The aesthetic response – the extent to which the practitioner can respond to the person with appropriate and skilled responses	Within each clinical moment the practitioner must grasp and interpret what is unfolding, envisage what she needs to achieve (with the person as possible) and respond with appropriate and effective action. The practitioner develops her therapeutic response by expanding her repertoire of available and effective responses. Habitual responses and routines are confronted for their therapeutic relevance.
The extent to which the practitioner knows and can manage her involvement within relationships	The practitioner must manage her own concerns so they do not interfere with seeing and responding appropriately to the patient and family's concerns (Hall, 1964). These concerns are negative influences such as prejudice, anxiety, stress, loss of concern. Hence concern has two aspects: a positive aspect of caring about or for someone and a negative aspect of being preoccupied with self. Whilst concern creates the possibility to work with the patient and family, it also creates vulnerability. Reflection is concerned with knowing self, even in its deepest darkest corners where much of behaviour is determined.

Contd.

Box 4.1   *Contd.*

The extent to which the practitioner can create and sustain an environment where being available is possible	The relationship between the practitioner and the patient/family takes place within a specific organisational and professional context. The practitioner may perceive many factors that constrain her availability to work with the patient and family, either established norms and ways of relating with colleagues, factors embodied within self or the finite nature of resources.

guide the way in which the practitioner sees and responds to the patient and family. As you read the practitioners' stories, you will sense the extent to which their beliefs are known and held. Use these stories to reflect on your own beliefs about nursing and health care and whether you realise these within everyday practice.

The extent to which the practitioner is concerned for the person

Concern might be described as the motivational force for caring. Benner & Wrubel (1989) equate concern with caring itself. They noted:

'Caring means that persons, events, projects and things matter to people. Because caring sets up what matters to a person, it also sets up what counts as stressful, and what options are available for coping. Caring creates possibility.' (p. 1)

Without concern, there is no possibility. In Tony's story, it was my concern for him that made me pay attention to him. He mattered to me deeply even in the brief moment of meeting him. This concern is so fundamental to the caring endeavour and yet, as Tony's story highlighted, it is a concern that was vulnerable in the face of my own distress. Like joy and suffering, concern and vulnerablity are a reflection of each other. The more I care, the more I suffer. The more I care the greater my joy. Unless I can sustain my concern, my self is threatened in my need for survival.

Concern for the other is not a stereotyped ideal stance to be adopted or a particular intervention to be utilised (Jourard, 1971). It is heartfelt and sets up the potential for involved relationships with patients and families. Carr & Kemmis (1986) draw on Aristotle to discuss the concept of *phronesis*, the sense of commitment within praxis as 'informed and committed action' (p. 46). Commitment manifests itself through concern for others, through the practitioner's self-challenge and effort to be effective in her work.

As a noun, commitment can mean 'a declared attachment to a doctrine or cause', although it can also mean 'an obligation undertaken' (*Chambers*

Twentieth Century Dictionary, 1972). From a sense of commitment, the practitioner acts according to firmly held beliefs and values about caring that implicitly lead her to consider every situation on its merits before taking appropriate action (Yarling & McElmurray, 1986; Packard & Ferrara, 1987; Cooper, 1991; Johns, 1993). Van Hooft (1987) examined the nursing literature on caring and noted the tension between caring as unconditional giving of the self and as a conditioned professional response to situations. He made the distinction between commitment and obligation.

Obligation is carrying out an expected duty. It represents the major ethical principle of deontology by which a person acts from a perceived sense of duty with good intention (Seedhouse, 1988) irrespective of the outcome; for example, the duty to always tell a patient the truth irrespective of the fact that it might be more compassionate to mask the truth or that it might lead to conflict with the patient's family. Commitment is the resolve to act out of concern. James (1989) noted in her research on nurses' emotional work with patients:

> 'Emotional labour is hard work and can be sorrowful and difficult. It demands that the labourer gives personal attention which means that they must give something of themselves, not just a formulaic response.' (p. 19)

This notion of *giving something of themselves* reflects the practitioner's commitment to act out her beliefs and values even in situations of personal stress. The contrast with a formulaic response highlights the distinction between the involvement or detachment of the practitioner within her professional relationships. Forrest (1989), in her phenomenological study of nurses' lived experiences of caring, supported concern for patients as central to a concept of caring. She commented: 'For practising nurses, caring is first and foremost a mental and emotional presence that evolves from deep feelings for the patient's experience' (p. 818)

Nurses often seem to struggle to express their concern for patients. The reasons for this seem to lie more directly with the conditions under which they have been socialised, rather than any loss of belief in caring. These conditions have not encouraged them to become involved in therapeutic relationships with patients and families. This understanding fits with Rawnsley's (1990) observation that: 'The personal warmth and affection of friendship seems alien to the artificiality of the legal bonding that defines the association between professionals and clients'(p. 46).

Rawnsley suggested that the word 'professional' needs careful interpretation and understanding when applied to nursing if nursing is defined within a caring philosophy. As such, *effective caring* will be enhanced by commitment and personal involvement in relationships with patients and families. However, the literature reflects a strong ambivalence to this personal involvement (Jourard, 1971; Dunlop, 1986; Menzies-Lyth, 1988). For example, Dunlop noted:

'Nursing sought to teach me to maintain both separation and linkage in my practice – separation "You must remember that the other is a stranger", and linkage – "You must think and act as if he were not". Thus one achieves something like "caring" ... a combination of closeness and distance, which always runs the risk of tipping either way.' (p. 663)

Practitioners who are deeply involved with their work express satisfaction. Creating the conditions where practitioners can become 'involved' with their work leads to more satisfying and consequently more productive work, an important consideration in a production-oriented society. Once practitioners are able to act out their beliefs and values of caring in day-to-day practice, their satisfaction is inspirational and seems essential to sustain commitment.

Consider how much your patients and families matter to you. Does your concern burn brightly or has it become dulled? In the following story, reflect on Jade's concern for Molly. Jade is a primary nurse. She shared this experience with me in guided reflection (Johns, 1993).

REFLECTIVE EXEMPLAR 4.1: JADE WITH MOLLY

Jade shared how negative she felt towards Molly when she was crying but had been unable to say what was upsetting her. Molly was crippled with arthritis and Parkinson's disease. Her failure to get Molly to respond to her interventions made Jade feel helpless. Despite Jade's impatience, Molly was eventually able to say she wanted help to get changed into her night dress before the night staff came on duty, which made Jade concerned about the night staff's attitude towards Molly. They had said that Molly was a difficult patient to nurse because she was difficult to help and took so much time. Jade noted her residual feelings of guilt which she didn't know how to deal with, but which she could clearly recognise: 'I knew it was wrong to feel like that ... I didn't like myself for feeling like it. I felt rotten about it'.

Jade acknowledged the contradiction between her concern for Molly and her concern for herself which caused her to feel irritated with Molly. Jade struggled to manage her negative feelings in order to avoid rejecting Molly. Molly's comments about the night staff sharpened her own sense of guilt. Jade noted that she was not skilled in this aspect of her work. As a consequence, she absorbed this distress and became distressed herself. She could not easily rationalise her residual sense of guilt because of her commitment to caring. Jade's concern made her vulnerable yet without her concern she could easily have rejected Molly on grounds of the 'difficult' label.

Nurturing and sustaining concern is a significant focus for development in guided reflection, enabling the humanist struggling inside to get out. My experience of working with practitioners within guided reflection informs me that there is always a spark of concern, even though it may be buried under a load of 'baggage'. As Henry Miller wrote in *Tropic of Capricorn* (1939):

'Men are poor everywhere – they always have been and they always will be. And beneath the terrible poverty there is a flame, usually so low that it is almost invisible. But it is there and if one has the courage to blow on it, it can become a conflagration.' (p. 25)

Miller's words are inspirational. If the practitioner's concern is barely a spark then I nurture the spark whilst exploring how the practitioner comes to feel that way. With Jade, I helped her put the threat into perspective whilst stroking her concern. Concern is vulnerable and needs to be cared for.

Deepak Chopra (1989) wrote: 'If I ever walked into a hospital and detected the spark of compassion had gone out, I could write the end of medicine – darkness will have won'. (p. 196)

Many readers will know from their own experience that practice can feel like a dark place, where concern has become dimmed by working in uncaring environments that have forced practitioners to become increasingly detached from caring in the illusion that they will survive better. In fact, caring is life sustaining and detaching self from caring only hastens the demise of the practitioner, besides increasing suffering for patients and families.

Commentary

As you read the practitioners' stories, consider the presence and significance of the practitioner's concern and the forces that threaten it. Reflect on your own concern. Is it strong or is it diminished? How might it be nurtured?

The extent to which the practitioner knows the person

'It is impossible to nurse any more of a person than that person allows us to see. If we permit him to utilise our freely offered closeness, he will not only let us see more of him, but he will allow himself to see 'more of him', so that he may, with excellent professional nursing, emerge as a "whole person".' (Hall, 1964, p. 152)

Hall's words lead us to consider the fundamental need to know patients and families in order to nurse them.

REFLECTIVE EXEMPLAR 4.2: GEMMA KELLY

One evening I wrote in my reflective journal about Gemma, a patient I had met earlier in the day. As you read this story, consider again the reflective cues set out in Box 2.1. How do these help me know and respond to Gemma?

The bell rang in room 4. No-one responded so I did. I realised that she had just come by ambulance from the general hospital. I knew nothing about her. She was clutching the bell . . . ringing it. She seemed confused, uncertain of what she wanted. A drink of water. She struggled with the straw with unco-ordinated actions. I asked her name. She struggled to reply – 'Kelly'. I thought this was her Christian name and called her Kelly.

It was difficult for me to respond. I did not know this woman and felt it hard to know how to respond to her appropriately in this first meeting between us in which communication was so difficult. But then so it should be in this first encounter rather than imposing on her a normative way of responding. My response could only be hesitant, tentative... tuning into who she was. I focused my concern to try to let her know I cared but I doubted whether she could read this message through her anxiety. I left her and the bell again rang. This time she asked for some food. It was lunchtime. I found Vera, one of the kitchen domestics, and took her into the room. She offered Kelly some food and talked through the menu.

I read her fear and felt her suffering. In response, I again focused my concern to tell her that she was not alone. I asked her if she had travelled alone in the ambulance. No clear answer from her. I wondered how she felt about being here but didn't ask her this at the time. I wondered if she was disoriented and anxious because of the transfer to this place of imminent death. I sensed this yet I did not directly ask her whether this was true. I felt this would only deal with my anxiety rather than responding adequately to hers. She was sitting on her night dress and as a result couldn't pull the strap over her right shoulder. I tried to help her but couldn't. I felt intrusive as a strange man helping this woman with her night dress at that moment.

I read her transfer note... no age or religion mentioned. She had breast cancer. Brain and liver secondaries... perhaps explaining the slight confusion and disorientation? I thought of her as being in her early 40s and felt sad for her in that moment. I read her name – Gemma Kelly. I felt a wave of irritation at myself for calling her by her surname. I returned to her as another nurse arrived with her food. She had fixed the shoulder strap! I really wanted to help her with her food because I felt for her. I wanted to help her and I couldn't at that moment even though I had told her that I would. The other nurse did not read my signs and I couldn't assert my need. It probably made no difference to Gemma yet I felt the other nurse was merely feeding Gemma as a task. She did not know Gemma.

Mary, the nurse in charge, said Gemma would not be admitted until that afternoon when her family visited because of difficulty in communicating with her. Maybe, but I felt this woman who had experienced so much was alone in this single room. No wonder she rang the bell. Perhaps someone she knew and loved needed to be with her at this time. The transfer might have been better planned. Mary said she was a 'nice lady'. This smeared Gemma's identity and I thought it a banal thing to say, sanitising her, reducing her to a patient who was nice, already imposing an expectation that she should be nice and that we should be nice to her. A gesture to defuse the emotional pain? Mary had allocated the new admission to herself but why, when others had more time to be responsive, to be with her? And, more importantly, time to be with her at this moment.

I felt very sensitive to who Gemma was, how she felt and how I felt about her. I saw her in context of the meaning that being in the hospice had for her at this time, linking to how she viewed the future. It was not possible for me to know. I could only reach out to her at the level of being with her, with compassion. A time would come to fathom her thoughts. I was reminded of words by Thomas Moore (1992).

> 'Day by day we live emotions and themes that have deep roots, but our reflections on these experiences tend to be superficial... not only are our reflections often insufficient to account for intense feelings, but we may be living from a place that is too rational and dispassionate. Rainer Maria Rilke advises the young poet to "go deep into yourself and see how deep the place is from which your life flows". We could all take note of this advice, go deep into ourselves and discover how deep is the source of our everyday lives.' (p. 235)

To know Gemma at this moment in time I needed to go deep inside me. I could have merely connected at the physical level but I knew her need at this time was related to her anxiety. As with Tony, I needed to know who Gemma was and what meaning she gave to this experience of being in the hospice. Using Newman's terminology, this required me and others to accurately read the pattern that rippled across Gemma's being. From a distance I could read the pattern she projected. I could use my empathy from nursing people like her. What was she thinking and feeling? Yet what did she mask?

Assessment

The essence of assessment is to grasp and interpret what is happening with the patient and family as part of an ongoing process, linked to envisaging what needs to be achieved and identifying appropriate responses. As you will have noted from Gemma's story, I use the word 'pattern' to represent the complex interplay of signs I need to pay attention to in order to know the other person in the context of the particular event. Barrett (1990) describes this assessment as pattern manifestation appraisal. Cowling (1990) more simply refers to this as pattern appreciation. Newman (1994) drew on Bohm's theory of implicate order (see Box 2.4) to suggest that the outward signs are pathways to deeper issues. By paying attention to the signs, the practitioner can guide the person to explore the deeper meanings of these signs which are necessary to make meaningful decisions about the future.

From a medical model perspective, this information has been centred around the illness or disease process. Nursing models such as that of Roper *et al.* (1980) have extended the medical model to include the impact of the illness on activities of living. The intention is to return the person to normal levels of activity. Assessment has generally been linked to admission, a significant process in the transition of person to patient. For people such as Gemma, admission is often a time of considerable anxiety where disclosure of self may be masked (Hughes *et al.*, 1986). As such, information may be limited or distorted.

Models of nursing, as generally conceptualised, tend to prescribe a reality of nursing that limits practitioners' imagination, creativity and reflection. These models encourage the practitioner to fit the patient to the model's structure, rather than being a creative heuristic to see and know the patient and his family from a holistic perspective. This state of affairs was evident when I reviewed the use of the Roper *et al.*, model of nursing at Burford Hospital to consider its continued appropriateness in the light of the hospital's newly constructed philosophy (Box 1.1). A strong sense of its inadequacy emerged. The model had become a task that staff were expected to do on admission rather than a continuous process that had real meaning or practical use.

Practitioners thought the model was an inadequate structure because it encouraged the practitioner to fit patients to the model, reducing the person to a series of systems, 'boxes to be filled in', often in a superficial way. The constant failure to adequately complete the boxes on sexuality and dying acknowledges the difficulty in seeing these 'activities' as part of everyday functional living. Sexuality reflects who people are. It is synonymous with the person's identity. Even responding to sexuality in terms of the 'sexual act' could not be addressed because of its social taboo. This was particularly evident when assessment was seen as synonymous with the patient's admission to hospital or health care. It is difficult to talk to a stranger about her sex life. It is even more difficult when the person being asked perceives herself to be reduced to some patient category. In other words, the patient cannot help but view herself as depersonalised. As such, she becomes effectively neutralised as a sexual being.

Undoubtedly, the functional approach has encouraged nurses to perceive models of nursing from a utility value or functional standpoint, often taking or modifying bits from models, yet this breaks up their integrity. For example, 'self-care' may have an attractive appeal because it suggests that a target of nursing is to enable people to be independent or to return to their level of *functioning* before the 'illness' event. Similarly, 'activities of living' suggest that this self-care can be packaged as discrete parts. Yet on a philosophical level, self-care must mean self-determination', being able to take control of one's own life in a positive frame of mind. If this is true, the focus of self-care on functional issues would seem misplaced because the functional would always need to be viewed within the meaning the 'illness' had for the person.

The physical self-care issues are symptomatic of a deeper whole concerned with the meaning and future of people's lives and the support they have to continue their lives in meaningful ways. The focus on functional activity may lead practitioners to fail to see the person and their distress at a crisis point in their lives. Failure to see and respond to patients in terms of the meaning and impact of illness on their whole lives is uncaring and contributes to suffering (Johns, 1998a).

From a functional perspective, 'self-care' is a deficit model rather than a growth model. The patient becomes a series of deficits that need fixing rather than being a person whose illness pattern is understood within the whole of their life. Focusing on the functional mirrors the medical model's primary concern with responding to and rectifying symptoms. It is a mechanical model that somehow dissociates the person's mind from their body.

On another level, 'self-care' might be viewed as a devious organisational ploy to shift responsibility to the individual patient, an abrogation of the caring responsibility. Even simultaneity models such as Parse's Man-Living-Health (1987), which are explicitly based on an ontological or existential level where the meaning the health event has for the person is the paramount lens for seeing and responding to the person, impose a rigid viewing lens on the practitioner. Johns & Graham (1996) comment:

'Models, by their very nature, impose a world-view that limits how practitioners see what is. In this sense models can cause suffering. Our models freeze-dry the flow of experience into a manageable reality, given our thirst to control things rather than let things be in themselves. Reflection [in contrast] intends to tune the practitioner into an openness and awareness of the human encounter and experience . . . and be a guide rather than an imposition, to free the senses rather than constrain them.' (p. 38)

The Roper *et al.* model is easily understood from a functional perspective because it seems to represent what nurses already do. Hence adopting the model requires minimal accommodation. Pearson (1983), in justifying the adoption of the Roper model at Burford, noted the way the model:

'. . . speaks to nurses in a language which is familiar and related to nursing in this country and hence its greatest advantage then is its ability to convey meaning to clinical nurses.' (p. 53, cited in Johns, 1994, p. 11)

However, it could be argued that its greatest advantage is also its greatest disadvantage because it fits in with what nurses already do. As such, it would not change practice. The outcome of reviewing the Roper *et al.* model was to reject it as an inadequate representation of nursing at Burford and to construct a 'tailor-made' model based on a valid philosophy for practice (Johns, 1994).

It is important to emphasise that Burford's philosophy for practice is the core of a reflective model, not a separate base for the model. Assessment is a process that is integrated within the practitioner's aesthetic response. Carper (1978) described this as grasping and interpreting the unfolding situation, envisaging what is needed to be achieved, responding with appropriate action, and reflecting on the efficacy of such action. Carper's aesthetic response reflects that assessment is part of an integrated complex process. As I assess, I am also evaluating the impact of my responses, even on admission. The way I assess is a caring act, responding to anxiety and symptoms such as pain. Assessment and evaluation are two sides of the same coin. Assessment is an ongoing process of interpreting information and envisaging responses.

Carper delineated the aesthetic response as one of four fundamental ways of knowing in nursing (Box 4.2). In this model, the empiric, the ethical and the personal inform and influence the practitioner's aesthetic response within any clinical situation. White (1995) considered that Carper had not paid attention to the contextual nature of knowing. Subsequently, White identified a 'cultural-historical' way of knowing that acknowledged the way all experience, and hence all knowing, is developed from previous experiences towards anticipating future experiences. Clearly, the way practitioners view and respond to patients is influenced by previous experience and the underlying conditions of practice.

Box 4.2   The relationship within Carper's fundamental ways of knowing within nursing (Johns, 1995c).

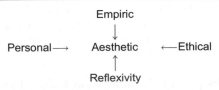

The aesthetic – knowing how the clinical moment is grasped and interpreted, envisages what is to be achieved and responds with appropriate action.

The empiric – knowing 'knowledge that is systematically organised into general laws and theories for the purpose of describing, explaining and predicting phenomena of special concern to the discipline of nursing' (p. 14).

The ethical – knowing what action should be taken within the context of the situation.

The personal – knowing self and impact of self within the situation.

Reflexivity – contextualised temporal knowing applied to new situations.

The Burford model reflective cues

The core assessment question the practitioner asks herself is 'What information do I need to be able to nurse this person?' To respond to this core question I designed a series of reflective cues (Box 2.2) to 'tune' the nurse into the philosophy (Johns, 1994). The significance of each cue is set out in Box 4.3. Over time, the practitioner internalises the cues as a reflective lens to view and respond within each unfolding clinical moment, transforming the cues into her own reflective 'working model'. The cues centre the practitioner into the unit philosophy and help her to tune into and know the person. As Meehan (1990) noted:

> 'In caring for a patient from a centred perspective the nurse is able to perceive the patient as a unitary whole... and be receptive to the patient's experience in the moment. Thus the nurse is better attuned to the patient and better able to communicate receptivity, compassion, and intent to help. Patients often seem to recognise this, and it is probable that this kind of attuning to the patient, is, in itself, therapeutic.' (p. 79)

To emphasise – these are reflective *cues*. They are not boxes that reduce the person into parts that require concrete answers. However, the practitioner may initially find it necessary to approach each cue as if it were a concrete question to answer, until she has internalised the cues as a natural (reflective) way to view practice. It is not easy to shift mindsets as previous ways of viewing and responding to assessment have been embodied. Lyn Sutherland (1994) noted:

> 'Although at first I did find myself going back to the Roper *et al.*'s headings to make myself secure that I had not missed anything, omitting what was physically important, I did not need to do this for long.' (p. 68)

Sutherland (1994) further charted the impact of the model on changing her mindset:

> '... because the emphasis is centred on feelings and the total picture of that person's situation rather than on their presenting physical needs, it forced me to move away from a need to find things out, fill things in and get things done as soon as possible in an orderly fashion. It forced me to start to listen to what patients themselves were saying was important to them and then to plan care with them from this basis... It gradually became a welcome release for me.' (p. 68)

Sutherland's words are helpful because she acknowledges the process of change and the need for support to move from one perspective of assessment to another. It is a radical difference that brought about a radical reconceptualisation of practice. It is not simply doing the same thing differently.

Who is this person?

This cue prompts the practitioner to see, acknowledge and respond to the person as a fellow human being within a human–human encounter. The term 'person' is an umbrella to cover all meaningful others within an understanding of 'who a person is', contextualised by the person's social and cultural world.

Box 4.3 The Burford NDU model: caring in practice reflective cues. The core question is 'What information do I require to nurse this person?'.

Reflective cues	Significance
Who is this person?	Focus on the person in context of family, social and cultural significance.
What meaning does this illness/health event have for the person?	Contextualise focus in terms of the understanding and meanings the health event/illness has for the person/family.
How is this person feeling?	Acknowledge that the person is potentially in crisis and distressed, therefore primary intervention to respond to distress in order to communicate concern and comfort.
How has this event affected their usual life patterns and roles?	Understanding the impact of the health event on the person's life/lifestyle.
How do I feel about this person?*	Acknowledging that self's concerns may interfere with seeing the person – monitoring self to be available.
How can I help this person?	Negotiating care with the person/other health-care workers and responding appropriately.
What is important for this person to make their stay in hospital comfortable?	Acknowledging that hospital is a major disruption and focusing on comfort and control to minimise anxiety and knowing that 'little things make the difference'.
How does this person view the future for themselves and others?	Helping the person explore the meaning of this event in terms of the future.
What support does this person have in life?	Helping the person take control of this health event.

* These cues have been developed from the original cues.

What meaning does this illness/health event have for the person?

This cue acknowledges that people enter into the health-care environment for various reasons. It guides the practitioner and the person to focus on the meaning this health event has for that person and to counter any urge to impose the practitioner's own meaning. The cue is the gateway to establishing the existential dialogue. It asks the patient or family member to reflect 'what does this illness mean to you?'. This cue more than any other enables the practitioner to focus and communicate her concern.

Empathy

Listening to the patient or family triggers the practitioner's empathic sense: 'what is this experience like for this family?'. Empathy is the practitioner's ability to connect with what the other is experiencing (Belenky *et al.* 1986).

In Box 4.4 I set out the factors that influence the practitioner's empathic response. I have noted the significance of the practitioner's concern in paying attention to the other person and the significance of intuition in knowing the experience of the other. By paying attention the practitioner listens and observes more closely, picking up the clues. The person senses the practitioner's concern and responds in more open ways (Hughes *et al.*, 1986). Whilst every situation is unique, experienced practitioners have developed their intuitive sense through meeting similar patients and their families and can draw on appropriate research to broaden their perspectives of the meanings people give to illness. Perhaps most significantly, the practitioner manages her own prejudices in order to be open to the experience of the other. This requires the practitioner to constantly check that her perceptions and interpretations are accurate within the existential dialogue. Heron (1975) warns about jumping in too quickly with interpretation – what he described as 'bucketing the wrong well'.

Box 4.4 A model for empathy.

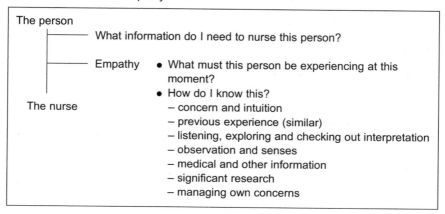

This understanding of the empathic response was constructed with Helen Hardy whilst supervising her undergraduate dissertation based on the Burford NDU model (Hardy, 1997).

I wrote the poem 'The colours of hope' after listening to a friend's story of her journey through breast cancer. I hope it adequately captures the essence of empathy. When she read the poem she cried and said it was exactly how she was feeling. How did I know? Indeed, how did I know except by tuning into her experience and drawing on past experience of knowing and working with women who had breast cancer? What does the poem say to you? Can you sense the woman's suffering and hope? Does this ring true for your own experiences with women suffering the potential loss of life and loved ones? The poem powerfully portrays poetry as a milieu for reflection.

The colours of hope

In this place at this time
my mind with colours rhyme
as reflections of who i am
in this dark place of solitude.

A dark place... i think of black...
seeing only a black hole
that darkens the window of my soul.
So i cannot see out and touch
my awaiting fate;
i strive to touch myself before too late
in my vain efforts to cope;
black... a prison for hope.

Or is it grey?
like these cold hospital walls
where the paint flakes and falls;
Like me my former glory gone.
Grey – like the woman's face across the way.
Like clouds on a gloomy day
that leaves no space for the blue,
and room for hope to shine through.

So i turn to blue...
The colour of my nurse's eyes
whose nonchalance belies
her concern for me;
i reach up to touch her face;
Not just another unfortunate case;
Blue – i sense the warmth of azure seas
and open my windows to its soft breeze.

I move on to red...
My nurse's lipstick makes me dread
my own self-image fixed in my head
as some mutilated being;
Afraid that others might stare;
despite my camouflage i feel so bare
i grieve my lost breast; shapeless,
no longer soft to my lover's caress.

And green...
to thoughts of fields of long grass
on summer days long past
with children for whom i weep
in the loss of their dear mother;
Can i give them hope of just another
Christmas day?
Where joy can rule and hope make play?

Lighter now... i turn to yellow
seeing the primroses, dried, pressed inside
favourite pages of books i cried
over in younger more romantic days.
yellow – the sun's warm rays
open my soul's window for me to gaze
across the landscape of my mourning
to watch hope's dawning.

White – the bright haze dazzles.
Is this God meeting me so soon?
Is hope already past the moon
on this journey into the unknown?
i am transformed and grow through this
ordeal
to know that i am real;
i sense my nurse's hand on me
and know not the hand of pity.

Eyes open to her warm touch,
a gaze upwards reveals her tender smile.
My children from the photo watch my trial
and test my hope in the colours of their
dress;
Caring, being cared for in turn
i find peace in this place in my nurse's
concern
To face me;
Hope inside me breaks free
as tears clean the window of my soul.

Christopher Johns

How is this person feeling?

This cue prompts the practitioner to pay attention to the person's affective
state, considering that illness may be a particularly stressful time. To tune

into the other person's rhythm is fundamentally an affective activity. This informs the person that the practitioner understands and cares. Until initial anxieties are acknowledged it is difficult to focus on other aspects of care.

How has this event affected their usual life patterns and roles?

This cue prompts the practitioner to help the person and family begin to review their lifestyle, reading the pattern for deeper underlying factors that have influenced the current situation. Often serious illness can prompt a dramatic review of lifestyle as the person and family begin to reassess what is significant about their lives. Understanding the pattern of the impact of illness gives understanding and control to the person. It focuses caring in practice as a health promotion and illness prevention model.

How do I feel about this person?'

Asking 'How do I feel about this person?' prompts the practitioner to pay attention to herself – to ask 'Who am I?' and to identify and manage her own concerns that may block seeing and responding to the concerns of the person. This cue acknowledges that 'who she is' is the practitioner's primary therapeutic tool. It also enables the practitioner to acknowledge that she is also a human being and that caring is a mutual process and, as such, is vulnerable to human frailties, particularly in the face of suffering and distress. These feelings cannot easily be hidden by a facade of coping.

How can I help this person?

The first five cues have created a clearing where the practitioner and the person can come to an understanding that care can be negotiated (as far as possible) and outcomes envisaged, prompted by the reflective cue 'How can I help this person?'. The negotiation is informed by reasoning, intuition, research, hope, beliefs, feelings, tradition and relevant cultural expectations, all mediated through dialogue. The intent is to set out a clear pathway for action by all parties involved in the treatment and caring response. However, this pathway is not prescriptive. It guides future understandings and actions as the caring trajectory unfolds.

What is important to help make this person's stay in hospital comfortable?

I always hear Macleod's (1994) comment ringing in my ears – 'It's the little things that count'. It is the attention to detail that communicates concern and is perceived as caring. Making an effort to say hello to a relative acknowledges and values that relative and informs the patient of your concern for her. Knowing what's important humanises health care because such things are integral to self-identity and self-respect.

How does this person view the future for herself and others?

This cue prompts the practitioner to tune into the person's and family's thoughts and feelings about the future. Such dialogue may raise many difficult issues and feelings, such as the prospect of dying or disability.

What support does this person have in life?

This cue prompts the practitioner to mobilise resources that the person may require at a later stage of the health event trajectory. In hospital situations, this is a significant issue around discharge. Exploring this cue may also raise anxiety and conflict within the family in terms of different expectations and obligations.

REFLECTIVE EXEMPLAR 4.3: MRS BANNING

Consider the way Leslie tuned into the person of Mrs Banning. Leslie is a primary nurse who works in a community hospital that uses the Burford NDU model.

Leslie: "She was such a one off. You couldn't imagine anyone like her. Her GP said she was an obsessive, neurotic and anxious lady. When she arrived here there was a look of sheer terror on her face. I had to respond. She said 'Dr Pressley promised me a single room'. I responded 'I might have one when it's free (but) that might be a long time or never. I don't know. You can have some privacy by drawing the curtains around you.' She said that she couldn't possibly sleep on a bed, that she had to sleep upright in a chair with pillows to support her back. I arranged for this and told her that Dr Pressley had asked for her to elevate her legs. She accepted this and put them up on a stool. She said she was in a lot of pain. I asked her where it was and when she last had pain killers. I offered her two co-proxamol at once with some cold water. She said she couldn't stand cold water and indicated to her flask of hot water."

CJ: "How did you feel when she said that?"

Leslie: "I momentarily felt put out but then I went along with the things she wanted in order to help relieve her anxiety. She also wanted a strong cup of coffee in her cup and saucer and some biscuits from her tin. I went to pour the coffee and she said 'I can do that, I am not helpless'."

CJ: "Did that make you feel clumsy?"

Leslie: "Yes, a bit, but I was happy to go along with whatever she wanted. I asked her what she knew about her illness, why she was here and what support she had. She said she didn't want to talk about it now, so I went away."

CJ: "You interpreted that as a dismissal?"

Leslie: "Yes. It was 8 pm when she arrived – she was quiet, calm, and grateful. She called me matron – she called me that all the time she was here, never referred to me as Leslie except once. She liked to be called Mrs Banning. She was very firm about that."

CJ: "Did anyone ever call her by her Christian name?"

Leslie: "I think one person did but she didn't respond ... reflecting on the consequences of my actions, I felt I did help reduce her anxiety. She was comfortable in her chair and she was surrounded by familiar objects – her biscuits, clothes, dressings, etc. She had arranged these things around her bed, with all her crockery, cutlery, newspapers, and books on tables in front of her and at the side of her. The curtain was drawn to the right hand side of her bed to make a private space. What's interesting about the way she had arranged her bed-space was it was just like a nest – during the time she was here she pulled the curtains back until they were fully opened and she seemed happy to be seen."

CJ: "Why is that ... do you think she had become used to the environment or was it her trust in the staff?"

Leslie: "Both."

CJ: "Did you ask her what made her pull the curtains back?"

Leslie: "No but I checked out that she was happy here – I reflected on alternative actions – I could have ignored her to get on with the other patients or got her to lie on the bed and to follow our instructions or responded with irritation to her anxiety, following the GP's advice not to show her any sympathy. However, the consequence of these interventions is that she would probably remain ultra anxious.

How did I feel when it was happening? I felt instinctively she was not unlikeable but her palpable tension made me feel concerned for her. I wanted badly to help her feel comfortable.

How did the patient feel? She seemed to feel more calm and at ease – my assumption was made from her appearance and non-verbal communication.

How did I know how she felt? She accepted my actions, she became quiet and noticeably unmasked her terror and pain, the way she arranged her bedside, her warmth towards me and Shelly [night associate nurse] on the handover walk-round, and how she became more openly warm in her responses to people, and her improved mobility – she could hardly walk or even stand on admission. Early one morning I noticed she had walked out to the single room to visit another patient. She didn't want to show the day staff she could walk.

What have I learnt? That responding directly to an anxious person's agenda may lead to a significant reduction in anxiety and allow the commencement of a therapeutic relationship."

CJ: "Did you feel you were rivals for control of the environment?"

Leslie: "In some ways – definitely, but I felt that it was more important she had control than I did. If I had tried to take control there is an even bigger risk that she would have discharged herself and no chance of a positive admission. When she came in I had the feeling she was going to go home and this wasn't going to work."

CJ: "Were you able to give the GP feedback about his briefing for her coming into hospital?"

Leslie: "Yes, but he was sceptical about how it would endure after she had gone home. He had a very laidback attitude towards her."

CJ: "Well he had written her off. I expect she knew that. How did your colleagues react to her?"

Leslie: "They found her difficult at times, and at other times had good relationships with her and responded warmly to her. Certain staff felt we indulged her far too much and we shouldn't allow patients to express and have their individual needs met to such an extent. These staff to some extent ignore the philosophy and the rationale of the [holistic] model."

CJ: "Did that threaten to undo the trust you had established with Mrs Banning?"

Leslie: "In fact, Mrs Banning threatened to report one of the care assistants. I felt more like an anthropologist than a nurse dealing with Mrs Banning!"

Commentary

Leslie was able to shrug aside the 'difficult' label to know Mrs Banning and establish the existential dialogue with her. Failure to tune into her wavelength would have precipitated an adversarial relationship that would not have been in anybody's best interests and would have confirmed the 'difficult' label. Clearly, not all patients will comply with the ideal patient role. As such, practitioners need to monitor their own concerns in order to to see and respond to the patient as a person irrespective of her behaviour. Where such behaviour is unacceptable, then this becomes a focus for understanding and negotiation.

REFLECTIVE EXEMPLAR 4.4: AGNES AND RITA

A significant issue in knowing patients is creating a space where the practitioner can spend time with the patient. Leslie noted that he had two new respite care patients, Agnes and Rita. He shared his experience of helping them bath and using this time to know these women.

Leslie: "I felt I got to know Agnes for the first time this morning since she arrived. I took her for a bath and she talked about her legs, the swelling and pain. We made frequent eye contact and she showed me she was enjoying the bath and was quite comfortable. She was crying out for Toby when she first came in. Now she seems more relaxed. She smiled at me after her bath."

CJ: "Giving you positive feedback?"

Leslie: "Oh yes. When I looked at her legs and changed her dressings she made it clear that she was pleased with this attention. After her bath I was helping her comb her hair, showing her the mirror, she said "go on, give me a kiss.""

CJ: "And did you?"

Leslie: "Yes. I think I perceived the 'stereotype' when she came in and now I'm seeing her as a human being."

CJ: "Did you check Agnes's self-assessment?"

Leslie: "No. I do need to contact Agnes' son and make an appointment to talk through this assessment."

CJ: "Doing this would create the opportunity to establish a dialogue with him and respond to his carer needs. Reflect on the philosophy of self-assessment in respite care." (see Box 4.5)

Leslie continued by talking about Rita.

Leslie: "Rita had a bath this morning. We talked about Burford and the countryside – the places we know. She talked about places she had lived, where her husband had died, her dog. Lots of personal parts of her life."

CJ: "Did you ask her what she was really trying to say?"

Leslie: "No I didn't. At times she just wanted to burst into tears. It was certainly grief she was expressing."

CJ: "Some people find it difficult to talk about their grief so they talk about all the things that surround their grief."

Leslie: "Umm."

CJ: "You didn't feel like going in there or would that have been the wrong time?"

Leslie: "I think it was the wrong time. She wanted an early bath to be ready for the chiropodist so she was anxious about that as well, but we did talk about the good things in her life that she valued. This was useful to know with her case conference coming up [for nursing home placement]."

Box 4.5   Philosophy of self-assessment in respite care.

- To acknowledge the carer's principal caring role.
- To minimise disruption to existing patterns of care and ensure continuity of care between home and hospital.
- To know the person's particular caring needs/lifestyle in detail.
- To know the little things that are significant to make the person's stay in hospital comfortable *at point of admission.*
- To understand and respond to the carers' needs (see also Box 4.6).

Commentary

By responding to Agnes and Rita as people – 'who is this person?' Leslie tuned into these two women and established the existential dialogue. All the reflective cues (Box 4.3) can be discerned within the brief dialogue. Leslie was gathering information for a case conference, highlighting the cues 'what support does Rita have in life?' and 'how does she view the future for herself and others?'.

By communicating his concern for Rita, he created the space for her to trust him and disclose deeper parts of herself. Leslie could discern the unresolved grief that lay just below the surface. He demonstrated his sensitive judgement in responding to the cues. Leslie noted Rita's different concerns within this moment; her need to talk about her life but also her need to be ready for chiropody.

Do these baths warrant his priority time? The bath is a significant activity within the whole rather than a simple task. The holistic practitioner responds on simultaneous multiple levels rather than as a set of linear tasks. Bathing patients is often viewed as an unskilled task for nursing auxiliaries to do yet, as these experiences with Agnes and Rita portray, the bath offered Leslie the opportunity to get to know patients although helping these women to bath is a sensitive gender issue for Leslie to consider because they are vulnerable. From a holistic perspective the bath is part of the whole, a moment of deep intimacy and sensitivity, steeped in ritual, a moment where the profane meets the sacred (Wolf, 1986).

Leslie noted some night staff were negative towards Agnes when handling her. We explored how Leslie might open up a discourse with his colleagues to both understand their feelings and undermine their negative attitude; for example, asking his colleagues directly how they responded to Agnes when she called out 'Toby' all night long. This attitude confronted Leslie with a significant therapeutic challenge: how to minimise the impact of these negative feelings on these women's care. Leslie needed to involve night staff in the assessment process to understand Agnes's needs.

In his next session Leslie picked up his work with Agnes.

Leslie: "I met with Toby, Agnes's son and main carer. It's interesting to follow up our conversation. The family asked to see me about lifting and the possibility for further [respite care] admissions."

CJ: "For teaching?"

Leslie: "Yes and for updating the assessment and for them to feel more supported."

CJ: "Do they belong to the carer support group?"

Leslie: "I'm not sure ... until the case conference I hadn't appreciated her daughter's real feelings. She had broken down and talked to the social worker about her relationship with her mother. Carers always seem to have to put up a front that they are coping. They seem uncomfortable about expressing any struggle because they are uncertain how we will respond."

CJ: "Do you mean how we might judge them?"

Leslie: "Yes, yes...who else is there for them to open up to?' There isn't a husband."

CJ: "Review the theory on carer need in the carer resource file. Note Nolan & Grant's research. They identified carer burden and the general inadequacy of the professional's response (see Box 4.6). Use this framework to reflect on Agnes' son's needs."

Box 4.6   Nolan & Grant's (1989) identification of (unmet) carer need.

- Need for information on a variety of topics from who's who to a more detailed account of illness and treatment and services available.
- Need for choice and some degree of control in packaging services to meet individual needs.
- Need for skills training in relation to nursing care, such as dealing with incontinence, lifting techniques, etc.
- Need for emotional support at a number of levels:
  (1) being recognised and valued for their caring
  (2) having someone to talk problems over with
  (3) help with recognising and dealing with emotional issues of guilt, anger, sadness, hopelessness and helplessness
  (4) setting the limits of care giving
  (5) negotiating responsibilities with the dependent person
  (6) some form of regular respite from their role as carer.

Nolan & Grant (1989) believed that lack of professional sensitivity may inadvertently increase carer stress and inhibit carers from seeking further professional help. This experience reinforced Leslie's reactive rather than proactive approach to establishing a dialogue with relatives. Leslie was challenged to consider his role *vis à vis* that of the social worker – does he hand over responsibility to work with the daughter? Role ambiguity can lead to conflict so clarifying role responsibility and role relationships is essential to enable professionals to work together effectively.

In his next session, Leslie discussed how Rita's discharge seemed to be vague.

Leslie: "It seems to be going in two directions. The daughter is the prime mover in looking at nursing homes. Jade [primary nurse colleague] thinks we should push her by setting time limits on her stay. That's quite hard but I see her point – there are problems with both the daughter and Rita."

CJ: "I spoke with the daughter [in my role as an associate nurse] the previous weekend concerning her attempts to find a nursing home, her history with her mother, and her feelings about her mother. Have you read the notes?"

Leslie: "I've missed that."

CJ: "Do you accept Jade's perception?"

Leslie: "Perhaps Jade felt the daughter wouldn't see any urgency in finding a nursing home. It feels like an official race between how quickly she can find a nursing home and how quickly she continues to deteriorate."

CJ: "If her condition is terminal, why push her into a nursing home?"

Leslie: "It's a dilemma as her condition changes from day to day."

Commentary

Within an existential dialogue with Rita's daughter, the discharge would have been negotiated. The potential conflict with the daughter reflected that Leslie did not know the daughter. The lack of communication and misunderstanding led to a potential breakdown of trust between the daughter, Rita and the hospital concerning each other's different needs and the conflicting perspectives between different nurses.

Leslie struggled to know how best to respond within this complex situation. Perhaps the therapeutic response was to give the daughter more support and utilise the social worker rather than put 'organisational' pressure on her. The reality was that beds were at a premium with a consequent pressure on Leslie to manage this resource well. Leslie's response was limited because he had not been informed of the associate nurse's discussion with the daughter. His failure to read nursing notes reflected a culture where nursing notes were marginalised despite being espoused as the primary means of communication.

REFLECTIVE EXEMPLAR 4.5: AGNES SIX MONTHS LATER

Leslie: "Agnes had been readmitted. I've been thinking a lot about her. She's growing old now, not wanting to live."

CJ: "Did she say that?"

Leslie: "She says 'I want to sleep – not wake up'. She's refusing food and fluids, says 'Don't disturb me – let me sleep'. Toby has been visiting a lot and so have her sisters. Her stay has grown from one week respite care to three weeks now. Toby is saying 'I want her home now' and then says 'can you keep her for a couple more days?'. When she had a urine infection I could justify that."

CJ: "The urine infection was the reason for keeping her longer?"

Leslie: "Partly that and drowsiness. That's how she has been going on. I think I have avoided talking to him about the future. The sisters come in and see me deliberately before he arrives. They challenge me about whether we are pushing Agnes home or whether Toby is asking for her to stay. They said she was eating and drinking well prior to admission which I know wasn't so."

CJ: "Did you point out that contradiction?"

Leslie: "No – I didn't rush in."

CJ: "You could see their motives though?"

Leslie: "Oh yes. I said she was old now. They were saying to me that she needs much more care. Toby said to Karen [associate nurse] that he didn't mind if Agnes stays here or came home but he didn't want Agnes to go into a nursing home. I asked the sisters why Toby had said that. They think Toby may have made a promise to Agnes. I said that Agnes couldn't stay here indefinitely. They listened to what I was saying. I said that it was up to them to get together with Toby about future care – it wasn't for me to act as an intermediary. They were looking for opinion from me to justify Agnes staying here. I felt the family wanted me to say that she was too unwell to go home and to tell Toby. I talked to Agnes – her responses were around her physical comfort and where Toby was. Beyond that it's not easy to have communication with her. The responsibility lies with them. I felt I could have been more definite with my view early on. I could have been more cathartic with Toby. I saw myself as advocate for Agnes."

CJ: "Did you give the impression that Agnes could stay here?"

Leslie: "I explained that she could stay here because of the UTI. The options were for her to set a deadline to go home or to arrange a nursing home."

CJ: "Have you involved the social worker?"

Leslie: "No, but she's on their books. She hadn't talked it over with me."

CJ: "Do you think that would be useful?"

Leslie: "I did yesterday. She thought the best option was going home and reassessing the support going in."

CJ: "She's already having a lot of support?"

Leslie: "Yes that's right but I felt I needed to get some sort of control for myself. I really felt the situation was drifting – the family were happy for it to drift without putting in any more support themselves. I feel I have avoided conflict and I must risk it. I tried to help them see they could have more care but if they didn't want her at home, I didn't have the resources to keep her here. I discussed it with the locum GP – she felt the best option was to send her home and reassess the support situation."

CJ: "Toby's dilemma – wanting her home but not being able to cope with her at home."

Leslie: "Yes, and the sisters can't expose this dilemma. She is going home tomorrow!"

CJ: "It sounds unfair that the sisters are giving you a hard time. Does it leave a bitter taste?"

Leslie: "I guess so. It's why I'm trying so hard."

CJ: "Do you think the sisters will go away thinking you are a hard man?"

Leslie: "They do seem dissatisfied."

CJ: "With the system, not with you personally. You are merely the symbol of that system. At least you can rationalise your feelings knowing that? Consider your relationship with the family and the relatives' response within Robinson & Thorne's typology of relatives' construction of relative–nurse relationships (see Box 4.7). The intent is to avoid disenchantment."

Leslie: "The sisters are disenchanted, reflecting the breakdown of trust between us."

Box 4.7 Robinson & Thorne's (1984) typology of relatives' construction of relative–nurse relationships.

Stages of development	Relatives' construction
Naive trusting	The family (naively) believe that the nurses view the situation from their perspective
Disenchantment	The family realise that the nurses view the situation differently – leading to conflict and breakdown of the caring relationship
Guarded alliance	The family reconstitute the relationship in order to get some of their needs met – they learn to manipulate the system to achieve this

Commentary

Leslie felt torn between the conflicting needs of Agnes, Toby and the sisters. Without doubt, the family was anxious at this pivotal moment in Agnes' life. Leslie felt he was the *advocate* for Agnes because she had no voice, except as known through some promise made with Toby that he would not put her into a nursing home. Leslie had great concern for Agnes ... and perhaps, as a consequence, he absorbed Agnes' vulnerable self and felt 'protective' towards her against her own family which entangled him within the family's interpersonal conflict. They struggled with the idea of caring for Agnes at home. They also knew of Toby's dilemma but could not deal with it. That is why the sisters projected their anxiety on to Leslie.

Rather than feel defensive about this, he needed to understand 'what meaning the sisters gave to this situation' and the full range of the reflective cues. The lack of openness made it difficult to know the sisters and work together to resolve this conflict. There was potential for chaos after discharge. Leslie knew he needed to expose the issue with the whole family, to be there for them to help them resolve their difficulties and plan for the future, mobilising support, etc. Yet his response was largely reacting to events because he had failed to establish an effective dialogue with either the family or his colleagues. Leslie talked of things drifting, yet this was because he avoided the situation. Ironically, his 'avoidance' only inflamed the situation with the consequence of poorly planned discharge and potential chaos and conflict with both Agnes' family and co-workers.

REFLECTIVE EXEMPLAR 4.6: PHILIP'S STORY

Consider the significance of each reflective cue in Philip's story that Jade, a primary nurse, shared with me in guided reflection (Johns, 1998a). Philip had dementia and was admitted with a chest infection.

Jade: "Philip actually seemed pleased to see me. He remembered, he recognised me, he couldn't actually remember who I was but he chatted quite openly with me which is something that doesn't often happen. And then we lost him! We eventually found him in the staff toilet. I expressed my concern for him. Mavis [the nursing auxiliary] was in mad panic running around the hospital saying 'We've lost Philip' but I knew he hadn't wandered out of the hospital. I automatically walked down to physiotherapy where the door was open. I knocked on the toilet door and said 'Philip, are you in there?'. He staggered out with his braces down and just laughed at me and he said 'Why?'. I said 'You gave us a fright and I wondered what had happened to you'. He stumbled, 'It's all right, I just wanted to go the toilet'. I said 'Okay, that's fine' and then walked back with him and we were chatting about why we were concerned. He just laughed and at the time I couldn't get any response out of him at all. It was strange because the whole of the next three days he was a lot warmer to me, whereas in the past he always seemed to have a masked face as if nothing was going on."

CJ: "Did that change the way you were towards him?"

Jade: "I don't think so ... no. I like Philip, you know how you just like people and perhaps he was showing me he liked me to..."

CJ: "You initially saw Philip as a 'dementia' rather than knowing him as a person. Because of that you underestimated his abilities and failed to interact with him?"

Jade: "Yes, the satisfaction came from interacting with him. I know I saw Philip as a label rather than as a person. The revelation is profound."

CJ: "Do you understand the relationship between Philip and his wife?"

Jade: "No, whenever I try to talk to her she'll talk about what she wants to talk about, then if it goes any further she has to go then. I've tried to contact her at home a few times to try and make an appointment for when it would be convenient for her to come and talk. She is always too busy."

CJ: "She's oppressive with him."

Jade: "Umm..."

CJ: "I discharged him."

Jade: "Did you?"

CJ: "When his wife was there... the way she bullied him got him niggled. You could really see him smarting every time she did it. She said he is quite unpleasant to her and I'm not surprised. She laughs about it, laughs it off."

Jade: "Umm."

CJ: "I think she must be a tyrant towards him. It might be worth exploring. You could just say 'How are you coping?'"

Jade: "Perhaps I could go and visit them at home or something?"

CJ: "She might have some trouble in dealing with that. She may feel guilty? Can we use my experience to focus on respite care not being a baby sitting service but focusing on carers and their needs?"

Jade: "It's quite often the impression you get from the carer; 'Oh he's yours now, over to you'. Its interesting."

CJ: "I get the impression that she may need some help."

Jade: "I tell you what I do get concerned about and that's getting out of my depth."

CJ: "My response to that is to get out of your depth and then share it ... yeah, jump in the deep end and actually find it difficult and make sense of it. My impression is that you won't get too much out of your depth and by being very aware of yourself you can say to Mrs Evans [Philip's wife] 'I'm having trouble handling this' – I would feed that back to the person I was trying to help."

We then explored 'jumping in and getting out of a jam' techniques to help Jade consider appropriate action.

In a later session Jade said: "Philip is back in. I have spoken to Mrs Evans. I saw this as an opportunity to run through things with her to enable her to open up with how she copes with Philip at home. She was always trying to get up and go as we spoke. She said she was going on holiday this week to the Lake District. When she comes back maybe I'll arrange to visit her at home."

Commentary

Jade had not involved Philip's spouse, again limiting the perception of Philip and denying Mrs Evans support and help with her own caring needs. Guidance challenged Jade to enable Mrs Evans to acknowledge that she was struggling to cope with Philip's care at home. Mrs Evans' reluctance to disclose this struggle told Jade that Mrs Evans needed to retain a facade of coping. The extent to which Mrs Evans would open up and respond to Jade's availability remained to be seen. Jade cannot help Mrs Evans without knowing her perspectives and knowing that caring for Philip must be within this context. Jade was empowered to speak with Mrs Evans, thus overcoming her sense of intimidation.

Within the existential dialogue the practitioner will come to understand the varying needs of each person within the situation and mediate any conflict. This may not be easy at times of distress when emotions run high and feelings are not shared. The practitioner may also find herself taking sides and 'advocating' the patient's rights and needs against the needs of the family. It is only when a caring dialogue has been established that conflict can be worked out in open ways. The family then knows that the practitioner understands their perspective and does care for them, even amidst situations of conflict.

REFLECTIVE EXEMPLAR 4.7: TRUDY'S STORY

Trudy is a district nurse. Her story concerns her relationship with Catherine, a woman with terminal cancer, and Gary, her husband. As you read the story, consider Trudy's ability to tune into and be available to respond to the conflicting needs of this family. Trudy uses the Burford NDU model to guide her practice. The experience Trudy shared with me extended over six consecutive guided reflection sessions. We had contracted to meet every three weeks for one hour although sometimes for unpredictable reasons, sessions had to be postponed. Consider also the reflexive nature of guided reflection, the way experience is built upon itself through each successive session.

Session 1

In our first session Trudy read from her reflective diary.

"Catherine is a 47-year-old woman with cancer in her bowel and peritoneal secondaries. She has a colostomy. Her husband called the clinic at 17.45 requesting me to visit. The message was 'wife unwell/colostomy blocked'. It was taken by another nurse. My dilemma – do I visit now or do I refer this to the evening nurse? I left it to the evening nurse. I rationalised this by thinking that it would be good for her to make Catherine's acquaintance. On my way home I pass nearby this family's house. I was feeling guilty that I had not responded personally, so I popped in. The curtains were drawn upstairs. Catherine was blind, confused, she had gone off her legs. She was lying in the bathroom. I helped to move her onto the bed and she then commenced fitting. Her two sons who were present could not cope with this. They fled. Her husband was shocked. She was fitting for about 15–20 minutes. I called the general practitioner, who suggested I made a 999 emergency call. I resisted this; I was asking myself 'do I want her to go into hospital?'. I didn't know the preferences of the family about managing Catherine's deterioration and eventual death. This had not become a topic of conversation. The GP arrived and gave Catherine some IV valium which worked although she continued to fit intermittently. Her husband decided on private hospital admission – we had to wait two hours for an ambulance to arrive. I stayed with her during this time. Catherine fitted again on the stretcher going into ambulance. I felt bad because I hadn't spoken to the boys ... was my decision to refer to the night nurse the best decision? I felt I didn't have the full facts of the situation and didn't know the situation well enough to make a good judgement."

I asked Trudy whether she could have rung the husband back to explore what was meant by 'unwell'. Trudy responded, 'Yes, I should have done that as Catherine usually managed her colostomy well.'

I picked up Trudy's comment about eventual death and asked her about her relationship with the family and talking about managing Catherine's impending death. Trudy said: 'I have known Catherine for seven months – she knows her condition is terminal.'

I challenged Trudy on whether she was avoiding talking about this situation with the family. Trudy acknowledged the need to manage hope and whether she should confront Gary's denial at this time. Gary was uncomfortable talking about these issues and for these reasons she had not pushed it. She felt sensitive about a right time to discuss Catherine's death and that this right time had not yet presented itself. However, she felt this event marked a crisis within Catherine's illness trajectory and that she would discuss with Gary the different options for managing this situation when she visited him on Friday.

I gently probed whether Trudy avoided discussion with Gary and Catherine because of her own discomfort. Trudy said 'My relationship is largely with Catherine. Gary has always seemed on the margins, seemingly uncomfortable with the emotional issues and focusing more on managing the physical. As a result I don't know him very well.'

Trudy continued to blame herself for referring to the evening nurse when she should have visited. I reflected the way in which, with hindsight, we punish ourselves yet helped Trudy to see that her decision was reasonable at the time, that she couldn't have envisaged the way this situation would progress. Trudy challenged herself, 'Did I want her at home for my own needs because I would prefer that?'

I suggested that Gary and Catherine had different and potentially conflicting needs. Trudy asserted, 'Catherine needs good symptomatic control right now but in a private hospital? I'm left with a sense that Gary just wanted her out of the way.

Taking Gary's perspective, I suggested that perhaps he could not cope with what is happening with her right now. Trudy acknowledged the point.

It was nearing the end of our meeting so I asked Trudy what she felt had been significant about sharing this experience. Trudy responded, 'Recognising that my sense of guilt is a reflection of a caring trap... thinking I should be there for my patient at all times. I seem to get entangled in these types of relationships. And secondly, my sense of unease with Gary that goes against my belief of responding to the whole family.'

Commentary

The caring trap, or what Ann Dickson describes as the compassion trap, explains that because Trudy cared she accepted responsibility for everyone's pain. She absorbed this pain as her own and suffered. She knew it was not her pain but could not easily break free from it. Her work was to balance her sense of involvement in ways she could manage yet without diminishing her concern.

Trudy felt the conflict of contradiction within her approach to Gary. She knew she was not available to him and that she saw him as a threat to Catherine and herself. He made her feel defensive and angry. I helped Trudy put this guilt, suffering and anger energy into a space where we could stand back and look at it for what it was, so Trudy could convert it into positive energy for the journey ahead with this family.

In this first session Trudy had come to view herself as if I held a mirror for her to see herself. It was a time of deep intimacy between us, reflecting her own intimacy with Catherine, a space to explore, know and heal self.

Session 2

Twenty days later Trudy and I met again. She shared how she had visited Gary.

"He said she couldn't possibly come home as she had a catheter, syringe driver ... a stream of problems. I struggled to respond to this. I needed to assess Catherine for myself so I phoned the hospital. They were reluctant to give me any information but they said it was OK for me to visit. Catherine looked really well. If she had been in an NHS hospital they would have sent her home days ago. She had no memory of fitting. She was no longer fitting but had massive oedema of her abdomen and legs. I was questioning her treatment with the staff. She was not on any steroids. I thought the staff had a very limited understanding of Catherine's drugs; for example, they thought 'nozinam' in the syringe driver was for the epilepsy. It was making Catherine sleepy. Catherine said she wanted to go home. She said this in front of Gary. I sensed the conflict between them."

I asked Trudy if she could have responded in other ways. Trudy was unsure: perhaps ask the GP to speak with the surgeon? I surfaced Trudy's anxiety that Catherine's desire to come home should be respected. However, I also reasserted Gary's perspective and questioned whose needs we are responding to. Do we understand and respond to him on his emotional level? Can he cope with Catherine's illness? Perhaps this is why arranging a support package for Catherine was not enough to persuade him to have her home? Trudy was uncomfortable but felt the hospital and Gary may be colluding in his best interests rather than Catherine's. We explored Trudy's options and their consequences. Trudy considered whether to involve Clare, the Macmillan nurse, more actively.

I asked, 'Do you want Clare to respond to Gary?'

Trudy responded, 'Clare doesn't know the family well whereas I do. I don't know how Catherine would feel if Clare came in.'

I challenged Trudy to consider whether it was time to confront Gary with the conflict of needs on the emotional level – a cathartic response to prick the bubble of tension yet to support him in facing up to issues he might want to avoid? Something like 'I can see this is tough for you, Gary'. I suggested that he might be feeling guilty about not having his wife home, so such a response may help him to face his guilt. It's not merely a stark choice of either hospital or home to die but to take each day as it comes, to leave option doors open.

Trudy responded, 'If she came home she could always go back into hospital or into a hospice if things deteriorate badly. I haven't really talked with him. I feel concerned that I would be manipulating him. I accept my sympathies and interests have lain primarily with Catherine.'

I suggested that a major issue for Catherine was to be in control of her dying, ensuring that those she left behind could cope without her. Issues about her two sons and why she needed to be at home.

At the end of the session Trudy felt the discussion had helped her to see things differently, most notably paying attention to the husband's needs and how this was central to getting Catherine home. She noted, 'It has influenced my future actions and helped me to anticipate what Gary may be thinking. I will arrange to meet him.'

Commentary

Trudy felt a deep bond with Catherine and endeavoured to tune into her wavelength. She resisted this work with Gary. Her family approach was splintered. Her beliefs were contradicted in practice. She knew this yet struggled to resolve her resistance to Gary. By empathising with Gary, I challenged her to see him differently, to tune into his wavelength and to understand his own suffering, to put aside her own concerns in order to connect with Gary, so she might become available to him. How do we sense what the other is feeling and thinking at such moments? Only when Trudy can open to herself can she understand and develop her empathic and intuitive sense and know herself as caring.

Trudy moves on in her journey. We had revisited issues surfaced in the first session and yet, just because we come to understand things differently does not mean we can easily change our embodied responses. Learning through reflection is essentially a holistic process of knowing and transforming self, rather than a cognitive activity. We are who we are for reasons that cannot be easily shrugged aside.

Session 3

Forty one days later, Trudy said:

"When I visited Gary and confronted him with the prospect of Catherine coming home he was uptight. He said 'I know I am being selfish but I've got a life to lead, and the boys as well. If Catherine is coming home then someone has to be here all the time.' He was adamant and said that he had to return imminently to work in Indonesia. I didn't pursue it because I could see it was making him more uptight.

I contacted the hospital. They said Catherine could be kept on insurance funding because she had a syringe driver which counted as treatment. I offered to look after her if she came home. But after that I didn't hear from them or from Gary. I became despondent about it. Then, this week, she was sent home for the day. Gary informed me and I went to visit her at home.

She was downstairs sitting at the kitchen table. She looked well. No syringe driver. No catheter. She was eating and drinking. Walking up and down stairs. Her legs were less swollen although her ascites remained and made her look nine months pregnant. She said 'I feel really well'. Gary interceded 'You're not well, are you?'. He was challenging what she can do, getting up and down stairs.

I asked her when she was coming home. She said she was working on it, pulling a face at Gary. He said that she was not ready for home. I asked her 'What can I do to help you when you come home?'.

And today? I heard that she is coming home on Thursday ... a phone message from Gary. The funding has dried up. He has got to come to terms with it now she's coming home. I have arranged a package of care for her. She's really determined. She said she had forced herself to eat to make herself better. There was no explanation for the epilepsy. They didn't do a brain scan and she isn't on any epileptic drugs. Perhaps it was a reaction from nozinam? She was on dexamethasone but not now. There is friction between them about her coming home. He is ambivalent about her coming home."

Trudy explored her feelings of involvement with Catherine. She knew it was going to be tough for her when Catherine eventually died. She felt that Gary's comments were offputting for Catherine. Trudy knew she needed to be supportive to Gary rather than confronting him because of the guilt Gary may feel about not wanting Catherine at home. This was an important development, to sense Gary's feelings and to consider the impact on him at a time he most needed support. I suggested that Gary might feel more comfortable if Catherine was being cared for within a hospice. Perhaps Trudy needed to confront Catherine with her efforts to cope and herself about colluding with her to create an illusion that she is more able than she really is, while acknowledging that was Catherine's way of coping.

Trudy acknowledged her resistance to and avoidance of Gary.

'After I last saw Gary, I let it go. I feel guilty about that. I saw him in the shops and I went off the other way rather than face him. I began to feel awkward with pushing it for her. Often at home I would think how she was. I couldn't understand why they had kept the syringe driver going. Her body is covered with abscess sites from the driver – they had to change the site every day. She's on MST now.'

Trudy reflected on how she had been drawn into an emotional web, entangled, and pulled between Gary and Catherine, suffering because of Catherine. In response, I helped Trudy to visualise and understand her involvement with Catherine and her other patients, using the nurse–patient relationship theory of Morse (1991) and Ramos (1992). Trudy immediately identified with the Morse category of overinvolvement: 'I have been over-involved in the past. I know that.'

I said 'You sound as if you think you should not be involved?'

Trudy: 'Yes, my ambivalence about being involved.'

Commentary

Trudy's resistance to Gary is still strong. Reflection is like a sculptor chipping away at his granite block in creating a beautiful image. Each action of his chisel is purposeful to create the image and through experience he becomes more adept at wielding the chisel. Trudy is guided to chip away at her resistance to Gary, by empathising with Gary's feelings and perspectives and challenging her own.

Session 4

Thirty days later, Trudy was 20 minutes late. She had been at a funeral that afternoon and then had to make a visit. I wondered if it was Catherine's funeral.

Trudy exclaimed, 'No! She's up and well. I'm seeing her twice a week. She has been having difficulties with her son. He has problems with drugs and also a recent court appearance because of stealing.'

Picking up the cue, I said, 'Have you helped the sons talk about what's happening?'. Trudy: 'No. Gary hasn't returned to Indonesia yet. He's saying he's got to go next month but he's also said that someone needed to be with

Catherine the whole time.' I asked if this was necessary. Trudy said, 'I don't think so, at least not 24 hours a day because if someone has 24-hour care she can't live a normal life ... could she?' I responded, 'If you're waiting to die can you live a "normal" life?'

Trudy said, 'Well, she struggles to do the housework but she can wash and dress herself, etc.' I said, 'You are responding to her in terms of things she can physically do. What about her responses at the emotional level? Is she coping at this level?' Trudy: 'Maybe she doesn't want to talk about this level. She gives cues like being "on borrowed time", etc. It's difficult to talk with her because her husband and son are often there and they don't want to talk about it.' I said, 'Maybe they don't know how to talk about it.'

Trudy compared this with another Catherine, who was also dying yet very open about what was happening to her and who needed to resolve issues such as who was going to look after her five year old.

I asked, 'Perhaps Catherine is ambivalent? As you said, she's not in denial, she accepts she is going to die but she also needs to cope. Perhaps because she does need to cope she's trying to be brave? Imagine yourself as her, dying – what sort of things would you need to do?' Trudy said, 'Well, sort out my children. Put my house in order.'

I reminded Trudy of the message from *Final Gifts* (Callanan & Kelley, 1992)' that the primary task for the dying person was to ensure that those they left behind were able to cope. Trudy again linked this to the 'other Catherine' 'coming to terms' and her actions. Even things like changing internal doors in the house – things she had wanted to do. She was now quite peaceful with everything sorted out.

I reflected, 'Perhaps we can see Catherine is trying to cope with chaos. Perhaps she does need confronting in order to help her sort things out. Perhaps you avoid this because of your own discomfort and uncertainty about her ambivalence. Trudy: 'I just feel with this family they aren't ready to talk about *it*. I don't feel her physical deterioration has become that marked where her dying has really become an issue. They are a "difficult" family, I have a number of people who are dying where talking about the death is not a problem.'

I took Trudy back to the beginning of our dialogue: 'All this came out of me saying was it Catherine's funeral!' Trudy: 'We have a lot of people dying – nine recently. It's stressful. It doesn't help having conflict with the doctors.' Trudy talked through her conflict with a doctor over drug dosage. She sensed she was not being listened to, yet Trudy had not backed down and asserted her point of view. Trudy said: 'She was short with me but she didn't bawl me out of the office.' I said, 'I've noted the "intimidating" factor – *being short*. Perhaps she was trying to establish a certain sort of relationship with you.' Trudy said, 'Some patients have commented on her manner – her new year's resolution is to be less short!' I said, 'It's promising she has that insight...'

We paused so I continued, 'Last session I challenged you to consider the balance of being challenging and supportive with Gary and Catherine.'

Trudy: 'My stance towards Gary has changed. I now see their relationship differently. I see that maybe he couldn't go to Indonesia because he couldn't leave Catherine at home and that being with her was an emotional rather than a physical thing. Could he focus on work knowing she was as she was?'

Session 5

Twenty one days later, Trudy said:

"I feel that Gary is now letting me in and that I'm responding to my intuition, that the right time has unfolded to talk about feelings and dying. Catherine is now in the terminal stage of her illness ... I went in following a phone call from Catherine that her colostomy was obstructed. Up to this time I had been going in twice weekly. She had been self caring so I went in to discuss what was happening to her. On this visit Catherine was in bed. She said she had great abdominal pain. I sought the GP's advice. The GP had prescribed a suppository but this hadn't worked and had since prescribed Normacol. Because of the pain I advised Catherine not to take this. I also referred her to the night nurse so she could get help if she needed it."

After considering alternative palliative approaches to Catherine's bowel obstruction, Trudy continued:

"Gary was downstairs during this visit. I had informed him that the colostomy was obstructed and that this was a sign of things worsening and her imminent death. Gary said it wasn't fair to keep her alive. Why were we giving her all these drugs? That we needed to put an end to all this! I asked him if Catherine was talking about dying. He said that he wanted to look after her at home and not to go back into hospital. I thought they might be strapped for cash but he assured me that wasn't the reason. She didn't want to go in and he had accepted that. The elder son didn't want to stray too far in case anything happened to his mum. No talk of the younger son ... he was still having his troubles. I'm now visiting every day."

I challenged Trudy on why she should visit. Trudy responded, 'Because my enrolled nurse is not good at counselling. She "whips in and out". Both Catherine and Gary made this observation. She's a good nurse but preferred going in to do something definite. I need to monitor the colostomy, to respond to the symptoms on a daily basis and to help the family pass this crisis ... continuity of care.' I noted, 'Being there for them?' Trudy: 'Yes that's right. I had two other patients who were similar to Catherine with obstructed colostomies. One lived for three months after it had become blocked. She would vomit everyday. In the end, faecal matter, not very pleasant. I have not told them about such possibility. Catherine is struggling to eat just a little. She had requested some 'HiCal' drinks to help her keep her strength up.'

I wondered if Catherine was hanging on to some hope and Trudy was responding on this level. Trudy acknowledged the dilemma of maintaining hope: 'I can tell by the look she gives me that she knows she has deteriorated, but she doesn't want to talk about that. She feels the lumps in her tummy, hoping the tumour will still go away.' We then explored the significance of hope and how this interfered with helping the family face death openly.

I challenged Trudy over her team leader responsibilities – what you should do when you know people in your team are not responding appropriately. Trudy found it difficult to tackle issues of potential conflict within her team even though she knew that such actions compromised patient care. She acknowledged my point but deflected the challenge to talk about Gary. We noted how tough it was for the onlookers to watch someone close to you die slowly and uncomfortably. Trudy linked this to other experiences where the person dying seemed okay about it but not the others. She noted: 'Gary is out of control, feeling helpless, very anxious and angry. He tested out the night nurse to gauge her response – which was okay! This is going to be tough, especially when she becomes more physically dependent, vomiting, etc. I feel okay ... not overinvolved. I feel happy because Catherine is quite happy. Things are under control. I enjoy visiting them. Before I wasn't in control.'

Session 6

Forty six days later, Trudy noted how busy she was and the pressure she felt under just now. She picked up Catherine: 'Catherine ... her death. She was fighting it to the end. She was on massive dose of morphine – 5000 mg in her syringe driver. She had a massive fit.'

Trudy read from her diary:

"I visited Catherine Monday morning early; the Marie Curie nurse had rung me to say Catherine had had a very restless night and was not responding to oral commands and there was a constant trickle of black fluid running from her mouth. I decided to assess the situation and ring the GP from her house. As I entered the bedroom I was shocked by what I saw. Catherine was groaning and rolling around the bed, Gary was trying to hold her onto the bed. She rolled from side to side, legs hanging over the edge of the bed, her catheter tube kinked and twisted around her leg, her tubing from the syringe driver had become detached. Clearly Gary was distressed. Catherine lay across the bed, her huge abdomen hard and contracting, her swollen legs looked heavy and shiny, her face, arms and shoulders so thin you could see her bones protruding. I sat on the bed, reconnected the syringe driver and checked the light was flashing. Gently I talked to Catherine, holding her hand. She was calm for a minute, then she began to groan again, vomited and started to fit. Gary and I rolled Catherine onto her side in the recovery position. I called for the GP to come straight away and rang the clinic, asking the reception staff to bleep my nursing auxiliary and ask her to come to Catherine's house urgently. While we waited Gary and I talked; I admitted to Gary that I had never witnessed anything like this before in all my nursing experience.

Catherine's strength was amazing, on occasions rolling on to her enlarged abdomen. All kinds of emotions were spinning through my head. I felt sad for Gary witnessing this, Catherine's loss of dignity – what an awful death and I was helpless to do anything. I had no Valium to stop the fit and no injection available to calm Catherine. I spoke to Gary and said that the only good thing about this is that Catherine doesn't know what's going on. The GP arrived – he was visibly shocked and passed me a Valium enema which I inserted into Catherine's stoma. Within a few minutes Catherine was calm. I asked the GP for another in case she fitted again and asked him if he had any midazolam 20 mg which I could use to sedate her as Catherine was very agitated and restless. He wrote the medication up in Catherine's notes and Gary's son went to collect the prescription. Ann, my nursing auxiliary, and I then washed Catherine, talked gently to her, comforting her, cleansed her mouth and put a clean nightie on and clean sheets. By this time Stuart, Catherine's son, had come home. I gave the midazolam 20 mg intramuscularly into her thigh and within ten minutes she was asleep. Gary, Ann and I all sat around the bed emotionally drained looking at Catherine. I knew I could not leave Gary alone. The situation was frightening for him. Gary thanked us both and felt reassured that he was not going to be left alone. He was happier that she was asleep.

What was I trying to achieve? My main concern was for Gary who looked distressed. Catherine would have been horrified if she could see herself, nightie round up her breasts, legs and bottom exposed, rolling around the bed, groaning, complete loss of dignity. Gary was distraught, unable to restrain her almost falling off the bed. I was frustrated that there were no drugs prescribed that I could have given. When Catherine was asleep and calm, Gary could manage and was in control. Gary very rarely touched Catherine – he always stood at the foot of the bed or sat on a chair. I never saw him sit and hold her hand although he always talked fondly of her. I came to the conclusion he was afraid and it would be less stressful for him if Ann assisted me in all nursing duties.

I've learnt a lot from this but I never got to grips with Gary. I said to him 'it won't be long' and queried whether he wanted her family present. He said they can come at any time but he didn't want them staying. He said 'I don't think of her death, I think of the future'. He never shed a tear. I went to the funeral. Her father was heartbroken as his wife had died of cancer as well."

I acknowledged the feeling: 'This must have been very traumatic for you. . . you moved a long way to accommodate Gary within your sphere of care'. Trudy: 'That's been my real learning to see and respond to the family. It's true, I do normally identify with the woman in the situation which often leaves me angry at the spouses, as I was with Gary, because he seemed to interfere with helping me to help Catherine meet her needs.'

Commentary

Trudy's story reveals her growing awareness of self in working within this family. Yet how available was she to this family? Her primary concern lay with Catherine. Trudy had tuned into Catherine, monitoring herself, yet still being drawn into Catherine's distress to the point where Gary was viewed as interfering. Trudy's dialogue with Gary was concerned with the attempt to shift his perspective to accommodate Catherine's, not responding to Gary in terms of his own needs. The consequence was potential breakdown between Trudy and Gary until Trudy could view Gary from his perspective. Then it became possible for Trudy to work towards harmonising the dialogues, to help both Gary and Catherine find meaning in this experience, so they could unravel the chaos they all felt. To some extent Trudy was able to achieve this. It was not a perfect ending but such situations rarely are. Issues such as supporting the boys were left relatively untouched.

Reflection was a mirror held high for Trudy to reveal herself to herself in context of the specific situation, peeling away layers of self until she reached her authentic self. In doing so she confronted who she was, her beliefs, her thoughts, her emotions, her attitudes and her actions. Trudy experienced the conflict of contradiction and yet revelled in her commitment to know and realise her beliefs about caring in practice. She discovered new meaning to being a holistic practitioner. Blackwolf Jones & Jones (1996) say:

'Perhaps you have already begun your path of change and are experiencing the pain of previous pains, as you open the cover to the book of your own life. The cover, which up to now had been carefully sealed up. Like the leaves of a head of lettuce, you are beginning to peel back one blemished leaf at a time, to reveal the you of quiet peace. Hidden beneath your polished presentation to the world, your injuries have been waiting for you to acknowledge their existence. It is time to view your injuries and feel your bruises. Through this experiential [reflective] process, we become real. We really become.' (p.22)

Trudy did not view herself as injured or bruised because such wounds were masked by the need to cope. Yet, as the dialogue revealed, Trudy's masks were gently exposed for what they were and removed, enabling her wounds to be tended. Perhaps 'wound' sounds dramatic, yet the metaphor of the wounded healer seems common to most nurses. *Who Trudy is* is her key therapeutic tool. Trudy not only made connection with her deeper self, she also connected with me, as her guide. In nurturing commitment, the guide picks up the practitioner wherever she is at. If the practitioner is numbed towards her practice, then this is the point of connection. The practitioner may be wounded and defensive. As such, the guide reads the signs and shines a gentle light to help the practitioner to see and know who she is. In an outcome-oriented health-care culture, the temptation may be to shine a bright aggressive light that frightens the practitioner caught in the glare. Remember, guided reflection is a *journey* of self-awareness and self-realisation for the practitioner. The practitioner must set the pace although the guide can always challenge this pace for its appropriateness.

Therapeutic journalling for patients and families

Consider any patients and families you work with who struggle to express their feelings about what is happening to them. How helpful would it be for them to write about their feelings? Would keeping a journal help them? Do such accounts enable you to know the person more deeply? Research suggests that reflective writing is a powerful therapeutic tool for patients and families (Pennebaker *et al.* 1987; Pennebaker & Susman; 1988 Pennebaker, 1989; Smyth & Pennebaker, 1999; Smyth *et al.*, 1999).

REFLECTIVE EXEMPLAR 4.8: MOIRA'S STORY – LIVING WITH MOTOR NEURONE DISEASE

Moira Vass wrote her story of living and dying with motor neurone disease in a journal. She wanted to share her story with other nurses, to help them understand what she was experiencing. Writing her journal gave her dying some purpose and enabled her to express her feelings of anger which she struggled to express to those who cared for her. She was grateful for that care but at the same time her anger dampened her ability to share her feelings. Moira wrote:

"I have motor neurone disease (MND). This is a disease that relentlessly destroys the nerves that enable us to control all our movements, while leaving the intellect and senses unaffected... There is no cure for this disease. I was told the cause was unknown and it was terminal. However, there is a ray of hope – the drug Rilutek. This is not a cure, but has been shown in trials to extend survival in people with MND. Its cost is somewhere between £1000 and £2000 per patient per year. Yet it gives the patient time and some hope. It slows down the paralysing effect. My attitude to Rilutek is if it does not cure then why take it? It only prolongs the agony and postpones the inevitable. The paralysis goes on unabated and death is by strangulation, a form of choking due also to the fact that the intercostal muscles are affected and you cannot breathe or cough. From day one I became slowly and deliberately *useless* and within six months I could no longer speak, eat, drink or walk unaided. Artificial ventilation via an endotracheal tube merely prolongs the suffering. Patients remain alert to the end and many need treatment to relieve their distress, as well as oxygen to assist breathing.

Living with tube feeding at home

MND affects the nerve endings and consequently affects the muscles in most of my body, but particularly all the muscles in my throat which means I cannot speak, eat, drink or swallow. I was referred by my neurologist to a dietician as the time had come for me to be fed by tube. My reaction was disbelief, anger and lots of tears. Then more tears.

By the time I came to see the nutritionist consultant, I had calmed down and accepted the fact that this was my only option if I wanted to go on living. The tube is attached to the gastrostomy. My reaction was despair. How can I live with this? The first thing that crossed my mind was no more baked or roast potatoes. No more predinner sherry, wine, all the joys of living. One of my favourite hobbies was cooking. Adventurous cooking, dinner parties, BBQ with the family, like any normal person.

The first feed was only 200 ml. at 50 ml per hour. The feed type was Nutrison and it was not a painful procedure. When the feed was finished this was followed by a 60 ml syringe of water to flush out the tube and give you extra fluid and thereafter a water flush every four hours, totalling 240 ml per day to prevent me from getting dehydrated – feed at night and water during the day.

However, it did little to calm my anger. I just wanted to stop the whole business and go to God. I could not see myself living with a Kangaroo pump and a plastic bag full of 1000 ml of Nutrison Energy Plus to be given overnight. The idea of the night feed was to enable me to be free during the day apart from the four-hourly water flush.

I laid awake for the first three nights in hospital, my anger only getting worse. Anger that felt like someone poured boiling oil all over my body. On the third night, I reached down and closed the roller clamp. I forgot about the bleep sound from the pump, which brought two nurses to the pump and they duly restarted the feed. They sat with me for a while and we had a chat. I was finding it impossible to come to terms with my new way of life, but I decided to take a more positive look at my feelings and especially the word ANGER. It struck me the word 'anger' is almost a cocktail of emotions:

A   Aggressive, to myself and the staff – zero tolerance
N   Negative thinking
G   Grief, crying, etc.
E   Emotions out of control
R   Resentful – 'why me' syndrome

So I decided, for the sake of my family, my husband but especially my three grandchildren, to make an effort because they all thought the feeding pump was a great idea. I made up my mind to come to terms with tube feeding at home although the sight of the tube at my stomach brought back my anger.

On Saturday morning, 14 February 1998, I was found unconscious by Gordon, who was unable to rouse me. It was decided to admit me to the hospice. I have no recollection of the tragedy. I came round with my grand-daughter Kerry, aged 16, crying, telling me to squeeze her hand if I could hear what she said: 'Please wake up Nan, we love you'. Twenty four hours later, I was awake to the reality of my condition. My living will meant they could not feed me if I went unconscious. As a result they were anxious to start the feed but I said 'No, no, leave me be'. By the fourth day I gave in and the Kangaroo pump and plastic bag with the 1000 ml of food was back. I was back to square one – I had to give in for the sake of my family.

Once I came to terms with home feeding I found it extremely easy to live with and having the feed at night was more convenient. You are free during the day to do what you please and go where you like. It is very easy to take a water flush with you. It took about a week to establish a routine. I would set it up downstairs in the kitchen, sit back in my arm-chair and watch TV. The feed takes ten hours to go through. When I am in bed I make sure the tube is free and to do that I attach the tube from the pump by holding it in place with sellotape on my thigh – so far it has never woken me up. As an alternative, it is by far the easiest and most convenient way. If you can still eat anything that is a bonus.

The Hospice

Following my admission to the hospice as an inpatient in February, I received wonderful care, especially as I spent four days on 'hunger strike'. To me this was the only way out – to stop all treatment, drugs and feed. The staff respected my wishes and while I was unconscious my living will [advanced directive] stated *no treatment*. When I regained consciousness I made the decision to continue cessation of all treatments. I found my family were devastated and my three grandchildren cried and pleaded with me. On day 5, I came back to earth to the delight of everyone. The nursing care in the hospice was a special kind of nursing but I would rather have had my rights and my way.

On discharge, I was invited back one day a week as a day-care patient. On the first day this caused me unbelievable distress. They collected me in a hospice ambulance; there was the driver, a nurse and myself. As my husband waved good-bye, I started to cry – another step down the MND road to death. Suddenly my anger exploded and I lost control, crying excessively and choking. The nurse told the driver to pull over to the side of the road until I had calmed down sufficiently. On arrival at the hospice I was taken into the quiet room and there I remained for the rest of the day. With their special kind of care and continuous oxygen for 20 minutes, I calmed down enough and fell asleep again.

I have come to terms now with the hospice-type care for terminally ill patients. I am going into the hospice for a week of respite care – the last week of the World Cup!

Care in the community

Learning to live with a progressive neurological condition, and in my case the advance has been rapid, has not been easy. Since my collapse in February on Valentine's Day, I am totally helpless and now require 24-hour care. The equipment needed to assist in my care has built up gradually over a period of time.

It takes one nurse to get me up in the morning, washed and dressed. I bring myself down on the chair lift. We found the easiest dress code for my needs consists of a silk top, slacks, knickers with pad, socks and sandals. What does break my heart is that I can no longer wear my size 12 outfits. Since the introduction of tube feeding my waistline has increased to size 16. The position the night team leave me in bed has to be the right one for comfort as there I remain until morning. I can no longer move in bed or raise my head. I was provided with an air mattress to prevent bed sores. My gratitude to the team. They always chat to me about nursing, clothes and fashion. I feel guilty that I need so much of their time. My particular hate was losing my independence, and in particular my personal hygiene. I found this added to my despair and anger.

It is times like this when I wish we had voluntary euthanasia. The patient should certainly have a say when and where. Life with MND is like a living hell on earth. Your whole body is dead. All I am left with is sight, smell, taste, hearing and sensation. Family gatherings and Sunday dinners have never been the same. I can take no part in family laughter and discussion. I take no part in the kitchen or the food shopping. Anywhere I go I must take the suction machine, my talking machine, a large bunch of tissues and a carer familiar with my management. Controlling the saliva which flows from my mouth is not only depressing but also embarrassing. I fold the tissue into 1" widths, fourfold deep and roll the top end down into a narrow roll. I put about three rolls in the side of my mouth since I can no longer cough, but if I have an occasional sneeze this prevents me from biting my tongue and my lip which is very painful. If I sneeze again within 5–10 minutes I hit the same spot. The surgery lent me a nebuliser to help remove very thick mucus.

Through Social Services I have obtained a wheelchair. I cried my heart out when it first arrived. Life in a wheelchair is a very different world. You feel so vulnerable and at risk. As the disease progresses I find waking up in the morning a slow process. My friend, the practice nurse, suggested 10–20 minutes oxygen is supplied. Someone has to open my eyelids for me – usually Gordon. The only way I can sum up this sad journey is with a poem I have written. What more can I say!

My living hell on earth

I walk alone
Along this path
Leaving life's hope,
Sorrow, love and pain
Standing at my gate.

I speak no more
I sing no more
I eat no more
IN MY LIVING HELL.

Sometime I wish
I could swallow,
But there's always
Something at my throat.

I drink no more
I kiss no more
I smile no more
IN MY LIVING HELL.

I see and hear
My world go by,
But reach out
I can not do.

My smiles have gone
I have no joy
I walk no more
To join my crowd
IN MY LIVING HELL.

I'm wheeled along
In my wheelchair
To a sea of knees
And a lot of pushchairs!

Some smiles I get
Some yawns and cries
Thank God they're not
IN MY LIVING HELL.

I tried to find
The peaceful way
But the road is closed
And I must stay.

Animals Rights have a say
They can die
When they say
Please God, why can't I?
IN MY LIVING HELL.

Reflection

Moira was very keen to publish her account. Louise, the day-care senior nurse, discussed this with me and I agreed to meet with Moira and discuss possibilities. I wrote in my reflective journal:

"August 4, I arrive ten minutes late. Moira is not there. Louise says she has been delayed because her catheter had blocked – will arrive in about 20 minutes. I am happy to sit with the group preparing for the day. Moira arrives. We move to a table. She is small and frail in her wheelchair. She has a piece of tissue coming out of her mouth that soaks up the excess secretions she can no longer control. She has her light speaker with her to communicate with me. I tell her who I am and clarify why we are meeting together – to consider her paper on motor neurone disease and ways it might be published. I had been strongly moved by the paper. I also felt strongly moved by Louise's experience as one of Moira's carers, with whom she had become deeply involved.

Using her writing machine, Moira tells me about her experience this morning with her catheter being removed. Louise has been asked to replace it by the district nurse. Moira says it was awful. I sensed this and ask if it was embarrassing. She grimaces. She said she could write so much more. I say she has written enough. Her message is powerful and will enable others to understand and learn. I pause and wonder what it must be like to suffer from motor neurone disease.

I say to Moira that I understand she wants to publish whilst she is still alive. I ask her 'How long do you expect to live?'. I feel my pulse quicken on asking this question yet Moira takes it in her stride. She says her GP refused to answer that question, but she expects to die soon. Of course, no one knows for certain but do we as practitioners avoid difficult questions? Does Moira's despair and obsession about euthanasia encourage us into avoidance tactics?

I understood Moira's need to write the paper as a testament that her life and her death were not without meaning. She had been a health visitor and a teacher. She said she had loved nursing and wanted to give this something if it would help others to understand. Keeping a diary was a therapeutic act for her. It helped her make some sense of each unfolding day. It enabled her to express her despair in the face of her own relentless physical disintegration and eventual death. The catheter was another marker along this road. A particularly devastating blow as it took away her pride. She had become incontinent. And she is a proud woman.

I asked her if anything made her smile – the sun shining in the morning or the sparrow singing. She smiled. She said she felt like the weather. It was raining hard outside. Indeed, she had shed many tears that morning. In her absence of speech she drew the tear lines down her cheeks with her fingers. There was no way anybody could take her despair away from her. There was no way she could rationalise what was happening to her, yet focusing on something positive did ameliorate her despair.

She was grateful to me . . . She joined her hands in thanks. I felt touched by this woman in this moment, privileged to sit with her and experience her dying. I was conscious that she, like other patients I had met and written about, were teaching me something profound along my journey to realise self as caring. When I left her, I sensed a lightness ... a soft spring in my feet. Why was this? Perhaps I should have felt burdened with her despair. But no. Indeed the contrary. I had been lifted by the experience, as if I had been touched by an angel. I felt a calmness ... a sense of humility. I felt that I was an angel, that I had given Moira some warmth and light within her living hell, as indeed Louise did. Moira nourished others ... comforted and cared for those who would care for her. She did not want to be a burden but sensed the struggle her carers must feel for her. She had shared her story with her carers ... when perhaps they had not realised how she felt and had been insensitive to her plight. They were touched and it changed their caring towards her. It had opened their eyes to what Moira was feeling inside."

Moira has since died.

Such accounts are priceless insights into the way people may respond to crippling terminal illness and death. The knowledge that her carers and society could understand what she felt, especially when she longed to die, was important to Moira.

Moira was able to express her anger which I feel certain helped her come to terms with dying and made it easier for her family and her carers to be with her. However, thoughts and feelings may be difficult to write about. A person may ask 'How do I write a journal?'. If so, suggest they start by writing down their most powerful feeling. This may make the feeling stronger especially if they have been resisting it. As such, writing the word is confronting and cathartic. Then suggest they focus on something positive about their life, either something current or a memory. The aim is to balance the negative feeling. When they feel more at ease, suggest they explore the feeling they have written down. Why do I feel like that? How would I like to feel? Can I share it with others? What would be the consequences of that? Do I need help? And of course, be available to help them talk through the things they have written. In doing so, offer them guidance, courage, care and let them know that they are not alone.

Chapter 5

Responding to the Person with Appropriate and Effective Action

Introduction

In the nursing process, the term 'intervention' suggests that the nurse does something to the other person. I prefer the word 'response', responding to the unfolding moment in an appropriate way with skilled and ethical action.

Ethical action

Carper (1978) has drawn attention to the way the *ethical* influences how the practitioner sees and responds within any situation (see Box 4.2). From this perspective, all action is implicitly ethical action. The model for structured reflection (see Box 3.5) explicitly acknowledges the need to pay attention to the ethical within the reflective cue 'Did I act for the best?'.

Box 2.4 showed the advocacy–paternalistic continuum that guides the practitioner to negotiate with the person/family where possible and where this is not possible, to make a judgement of what is best, based on paternalistic criteria. Central to these criteria is the concept of autonomy. Ethical principles exist to guide what's best within any society. Yet what is best cannot be prescribed, it must always be interpreted within the particular situation. As such, ethical decision making takes place within a tension between ethical principles and the ethic of the situation (Cooper, 1991). Decision making can never be a rational formulaic response because every human encounter of suffering is unique. Emotions energise the ethical quest (Callahan, 1988) and hence the need for the practitioner to know herself in order to make good ethical decisions. Ethical action does not necessarily follow knowing what's best in terms of professional interests. Seedhouse's ethical grid (1988) and Ferrell's model for ethical decision making (1998) offer useful frameworks in which to consider and reflect on appropriate responses.

REFLECTIVE EXEMPLAR 5.1: WILLIAM

Consider the ethical dimensions of caring within my reflective account of working with William one morning in the hospice. Consider also the significance of knowing him and understanding his perspective.

William is 66, an American living in England with his English wife. I asked, 'Shall I call you William?' He said 'Yes, not Willy. I don't like the connotation.' We laughed. He says he endures England because his wife wishes to be here, yet the climate is not conducive to his severe arthritis. He talked fondly of his home in Kansas and, given the choice of where to live, would prefer to be there. He mentioned his three sons, one who lives in England whom he sees every few months and two who live in Texas and whom he sees every few years. A rueful smile.

I sensed the family were not close and relationships between him and his wife were in crisis at this pivotal point in his health experience, reflected in the tension about his return home, mentioned in the social support person's notes. He did not disclose this in conversation; in fact, he did not denigrate his wife at all. Perhaps he endured because he was now so powerless and helpless in the face of his future.

The main focus of the conversation concerned his arthritis. He talked about his recent surgery 18 months ago to his right knee, resulting in considerable trauma and skin graft. The result was massive deformity and lack of movement. Besides arthritis, he had also been diagnosed to have cancer of the lung, yet the arthritis was his concern. The lungs were apparently unsymptomatic. I had seen no evidence of any treatment for his cancer within the notes. It was not mentioned in our conversation.

When he had come to the hospice for rehabilitation he had been very stiff with early signs of pressure sores to both heels and sacral area. He was bothered by the smell of his wounds. Indeed, the smell pervaded the environment. As I sit here, many hours later, I can smell this as if it had pervaded my own being. I wondered if incense might help. Chlöe said she used aromatherapy with lemon grass and that she did do some massage with William, usually in the afternoon. I did not push the issue of the smell that bothered him but it may have been possible to be more proactive in responding to this problem.

During the progress of his wash, Chlöe dressed the wounds, noting the rapid deterioration of the sacral wounds. Her approach lacked aseptic vigilance but she rationalised this as the wound was already infected. William cried out as the Kaltostat packing was pushed in. I thought that perhaps the pain might have been anticipated and breakthrough analgesia planned, although said nothing at this time in front of William because I did not want to criticise and antagonise Chlöe.

Despite the extent of his tissue damage, William had rejected a Pegasus mattress because he found the mattress movement caused him much pain during the night. He remarked 'It was as if the pain dug deep within me'. He just had a Spenco mattress. He sat in a chair, where likewise he had discarded the Roho cushion for an egg box. With much effort he stood and walked, easing the sacral pressure and exercising his stiffened joints. He said 'I need to do more of this'. He noted the severe pain of the arthritis and the difficulty in controlling this. He had a considerable dosage of ibuprofen and MST and yet this pain remained poorly controlled. He was not prepared to endure the arthritis and sit passively to avoid pain. He had a life still to live! William said he did not get bored in the room, resisting the suggestion to sit in another environment. He seemed contained, managing to keep a lid on the conflicts within his life; indeed, being positive when the future looked so bleak.

William said he was going home on Thursday but I could see him being admitted to a general hospital soon after because of his pressure sore deterioration. I wondered if by Thursday he would even be able to go home despite the support package. I prompted a discussion of William's care at coffee. This evoked strong opinions about whether to let him make the decision about his comfort at the cost of the pressure area development. Should he be confronted with his decision? Chlöe felt that this was his decision and that it should be respected. Yet was his decision well enough informed? Should he be confronted with the consequences of his decision? What were his motives behind disregarding advice? Perhaps other alternatives might be explored, for example a Clinitron bed. The costs were noted as prohibitive. Yet at what cost the consequences? Chlöe's was the alternative voice. There was a genuine acceptance of her point of view, her paternalistic act to enable William's voice to be heard within this forum. The consensus opinion was that William should be confronted and even have the pressure treatment imposed.

Yet this forum was not making this decision. Where the nexus of authority to make this decision lay was not clear to me. Does it lie with each nurse allocated to William? Was it raised at the handover? It wasn't and neither was the dilemma reflected in his notes. Was it raised on the ward round and the decision deferred to medical authority? No. I am tempted to anticipate the outcome of this turn of events but refrain.

I asked myself How do I feel about William?' I felt quite detached from him, almost indifferent to him except when I combed his hair. Then I felt for him. Perhaps I was slightly irritated with him because I could see what would inevitably happen to him with his sores. Did he know this, I wonder? I felt the issue was avoided, that his perspective was too readily complied with. The lack of continuity of care impacts negatively on his care. Chlöe is allocated today; who tomorrow? This discontinuity was reflected through the notes of the unfolding shifts. Nurses pick him up and put him down again. The continuity was fragmented. He was fragmented.

No-one knew him well enough and who had penetrated who he really was? On the surface he was easy to talk with; his deeper self was contained and perhaps that was the reason I felt detached from him.

On reading William's notes, I was struck by the inadequacy of the nursing process notes regarding his care. They told me little meaningful or practical about him. The smell and pain of the wound and wound dressing were not mentioned and even the technical care of his wounds was inadequately stated. When I casually mentioned to Chlöe the use of mapping techniques for his wounds I felt a tenseness, a defence against a criticism which silenced me in the moment. I felt that staff minimised the 'technical' to promote the 'palliative'. A strange feeling. Neither was Chlöe's aromatherapy work documented. Was this merely some periph-eral activity that was not worth mentioning?

I did not write in the notes but perhaps I should have done. But these were not my patients and I did not feel invited to write. I would also have liked to have been with the doctor as he visited these patients this after-noon. He went with the nurse in charge, her information gleaned during the handover from Chlöe and from accumulated oral knowing. Perhaps I could have insisted on being there, as might have Chlöe. But we didn't. Culture is a powerful barrier to asserting self. William's smell was the core of his experience. It most concerned him and most concerned us. The smell symbolised his predicament ... his spiritual decay reflected in his physical decay.

Ethical mapping

William's story is riddled with dilemmas and questions. How does he view the future? What are his needs? How should we best respond to him? Consider three dilemmas.

(1) Should the care team confront and assert their view of the best response to his wounds?
(2) Should the wound dressing be done with more aseptic vigilance during the wash?
(3) Should we offer aromatherapy as a continual therapeutic response?

To help practitioners respond to the MSR cue 'Did I act for the best?', I developed ethical mapping (Box 5.1). I have inserted the two dilemmas into the equation.

'Ethical mapping guides the practitioner to view the various perspectives and contextual factors within any ethical decision. At each point within this "map", the supervisor challenges the practitioner to understand and balance the dynamics towards making the 'right' decision in the particular circumstance. The map helps

Box 5.1   Ethical grid for considering dilemmas (Johns, 1998c 1999a).

Patient's/family's perspective	Who has AUTHORITY TO ACT?	Doctor's perspective
Is there CONFLICT OF VALUES between perspectives?	**The situation/dilemma** (1) Should we offer aromatherapy as a continual therapeutic response? (2) Should the care team assert their view of the best response to his wound?	How do ETHICAL PRINCIPLES inform this situation? ● Autonomy ● Do no harm ● Truth telling ● The greatest good ● Duty
Nurse(s)' perspectives	How was the decision actually made in terms of POWER RELATIONSHIPS?	Organisation's perspective

the practitioner "see" the different and often contradictory perspectives of any situation, and to examine the factors that determine which perspective prevails. The grid helps the practitioner to focus on the conflict of values and power relationships that exist within the Unit and which largely determine who makes the decision.

From a reflective perspective, ethical principles, like all extant sources of knowledge, exist only to inform the practitioner. They cannot prescribe what is best, at least not without defying the particular circumstance. Often ethical principles are contradictory; truth telling may be harmful; respecting autonomy may lead to conflict concerning who makes the decision over what's best. The consideration of power dynamics guides the practitioner to explore whose authority determines the decision to act within the particular situation. The intention is to help the practitioner understand and expand their own boundaries for making decision's vis-à-vis others in terms of achieving caring.' (Johns, 1999a)

I have inserted a number of key ethical principles within the grid for the reader's consideration. Seedhouse (1988) is very persuasive in asserting that the highest ethical principle is respecting and creating the opportunity for the patient to exercise autonomy. Clearly, William was able to consider his best interests despite the obvious consequence of doing himself harm by objecting to certain wound care choices. Within a hospice philosophy, cure not being the primary viewing lens made his views more acceptable. However, many nurses felt uncomfortable with this state of affairs. The practitioner's duty was to confront him, give information, offer choices and help him (and his family) explore the consequences of his decisions; this is the existential dialogue. The authority for making the decision lay with him. In more acute settings, the doctor's perspective may be more influential.

Should Chlöe have done the wound dressing in a clean rather than aseptic fashion? Her argument was that the wound was already dirty. However, she wanted to finish William and move on to another patient. For whose benefit was this action performed or did it lead to mutual benefit? Was William prepared well enough for the dressing? At Burford we deconstructed all tasks. As such, a wound would have been dressed following the wash, as Chlöe had done. However, this needed to be a reflective action rather than simply getting something done.

The dilemma of aromatherapy is a very different situation. William clearly benefited from aromatherapy and looked forward to his sessions with Chlöe. Indeed, he felt a strong connection with her because of this. Use of time, for example for Chlöe to use aromatherapy within the particular situation, is always an ethical issue. How best to use time? What is the greatest priority? If I spend more time with William now, will it disadvantage another patient or family? Use of time requires a constant interpretation of multiple situations within the principle of greatest good. However, Chlöe might have burnt some incense to neutralise the smell. This would not have taken time. She had simply got locked into a habitual pattern of doing this therapy in the afternoons. Hence I should have been more assertive and confronted her restrictive action to benefit William. I compensated by raising it at a staff meeting to prompt a review of treatment and exploration of feelings.

This reflects the way ethical action is often compromised because of a greater need to avoid conflict, usually concerned with status and power. As a consequence, the patient's or family's needs are sacrificed.

Responding with appropriate and effective action

William's story reflects the aesthetic response, the way the reflective practitioner:

- grasps and interprets the situation;
- envisages and negotiates (as able) the therapeutic outcome(s);
- responds with the most appropriate and (hopefully) skilled action;
- reflects to determine the efficacy of the action and subsequently to learn through the situation to inform future situations.

The practitioner must always accept responsibility for ensuring the adequacy of her responses. To achieve this, the practitioner is an active creator of her own practice, constantly striving to become more effective and, in doing so, to expand her repertoire of available interventions to work with the person and family. Practitioners locked into hierarchical organisational models lacking this sense of personal autonomy or authority may find this difficult. At Burford, we funded a care assistant to undertake a massage and aroma-therapy course to become a resource for staff and patients. Other examples of appropriate and innovative responses are using therapeutic touch, visuali-sation and guided imagery (Madrid, 1990; Meehan, 1990; Sayre-Adams & Wright, 1995). However. these therapies need to be introduced with caution in order to ensure safety, consistency, continuity and efficacy.

Heron

John Heron's six-category intervention analysis (1975) offers a particularly useful framework for practitioners to view appropriate ways of responding within intended therapeutic relationships (Box 5.2). Burnard and Morrison (1991) undertook a small study that illustrated that nurses avoided using confrontation, catharsis and catalytic type responses and preferred giving advice and information and being supportive. They considered how catalytic, cathartic and confronting approaches involved an 'investment of self' which may be emotionally draining for the practitioner. Yet these are the very types of responses necessary to work within a holistic perspective. Nurses had not been prepared to use these types of responses. The reflective cue 'How is this person feeling?' requires a cathartic response; for example 'How are you feeling?' or 'I can see this is difficult for you?'.

Box 5.2   Heron's six-category intervention analysis (1975).

Giving information – Drawing on technical knowledge to help inform the person to make a good decision
Giving advice – Sharing an opinion to help the person see other perspectives
Confrontation – Challenging the person's restricted beliefs, attitudes or behaviour
Being cathartic – Enabling the person to express some emotion
Being catalytic – Enabling the person to talk through an issue
Being supportive – Communicating concern and being available

Nurses seem concerned about 'getting in too deep' and not knowing how to take the dialogue forward. A good illustration is offered by Caitlin when she avoided talking to the spouse of a dying man. After guided reflection Caitlin did engage the spouse, who began to cry. As Caitlin put it 'Oh Lord, I've delved in to it now' (Johns, 1997b). As a consequence, Caitlin became available to the spouse.

Confrontation often seems to be equated with conflict and the antithesis of caring. Heron (1975) defined confrontation as a therapeutic action – to challenge the restricted beliefs, attitudes or actions of the other person. To be effective, confrontation requires a clear therapeutic focus within a trusting relationship, when the person knows the practitioner is concerned. The consequence may be uncomfortable for both the patient and practitioner. If so, the discomfort is another cue for the practitioner to respond to – 'I can see this is uncomfortable for you?'. I term this type of response 'pricking the bubble' – to expose and deal with tension as it arises rather than letting it become a source of relational breakdown.

REFLECTIVE EXEMPLAR 5.1: KAREN WORKING WITH MRS KITCHEN

Consider the experience Karen shared with me within guided reflection concerning confronting Mrs Kitchen. This was shared in session 8, six months after Karen commenced work on the unit as an associate nurse in her first post since qualifying.

Karen: "Because it's quiet I've been able to spend time sitting, being with patients, to the point that I found I could challenge the behaviour of one patient. It didn't feel like I had ever done that before – it felt really good. Mrs Kitchen is a very independent 93-year-old lady who had a 'dynamic hip screw'. She was transferred from a general hospital for postoperative rehabilitation. Now she wants to get home but is relying heavily on her zimmer frame, not using her sticks. So I challenged her and said if she wants to be as independent as she was prior to the accident then why was she holding herself back? It seemed really funny, she hadn't thought about it, hadn't realised it at all."

CJ: "So how did she respond?"

Karen: "A lot better than I thought. I thought she would withdraw or retaliate, fight back. But she was thoughtful for a couple of minutes and then she agreed with me. She could see it."

CJ: "Did it change her behaviour?"

Karen: "She was more determined to try the sticks."

CJ: "But?"

Karen: "She still uses the zimmer frame."

CJ: "Have you given her that feedback?"

Karen: "No, not yet. I've been working a lot of late shifts recently. She says she's tired, and that she has used them in the morning."

CJ: "You accept that from her?"

Karen: "I have done. I came to work today thinking I'm going to get her going again tonight."

CJ: "For your benefit or hers?"

Karen: "Both of us, but certainly for me. I want to follow through the good I feel I'm doing."

CJ: "And for her?"

Karen: "She obviously wants to be independent again."

CJ: "Do you think she's giving you two messages?"

Karen thought about this: "She's saying she wants to be independent but she's a bit frightened and scared of it."

CJ: "Have you tried talking to her about the accident? She may have repressed this, which is now affecting her confidence. Can you relate this experience to Elizabeth?"

Karen: "No. What do you mean?"

CJ: "Your difficulty in challenging her. You thought you would get a negative response. You associated confrontation with conflict, and your wish to avoid conflict?"

Karen: "Because I did challenge her, maybe I did subconsciously learn from that last session."

CJ: "How did you feel when you gave her that feedback?"

Karen: "I felt quite strong. It was only after I said it that I thought should I have said that."

CJ: "And you challenged yourself because?"

Karen: "I suppose because I had never done it so directly before, and I wondered whether I was being too blunt."

CJ: "So you learnt you were not too blunt and that challenging can be a positive thing. View confrontation within Heron's six-category intervention analysis." (Box 5.2)

Karen felt uncertain and unskilled in using cathartic and confrontation interventions. However, she said she would confront Mrs Kitchen that evening. I shared with Karen a pattern I had analysed using Heron's framework.

- When an underlying emotion is sensed' use a cathartic response – 'You seem afraid to use your sticks.' 'You seem angry at my insistence you should walk with your sticks.' The intention is to get the emotion expressed so that it can be released.
- Then use a catalytic response to help the person talk through the issues in order to find meaning in the emotion and understand deeper underlying reasons for behaviour.
- Confrontation can then be used to challenge yet always within a supportive framework of the existential dialogue established through the cathartic and catalytic responses. It is perverse for Karen to use confrontation in response to her concerns; for example, frustration at Mrs Kitchen's lack of progress.

We rehearsed how Karen might use these interventions that evening.

Karen continued: "The thing I was worrying about was, that as an associate nurse I might be tripping over boundaries and challenging Gayle.
CJ: "Can you answer that question yourself?"
Karen: "I'm torn over this. Half of me says I was there at the time and was right to do this, whilst the other half of me says I don't know. I haven't shared it with Gayle. There is no obvious place in the notes to write this. Gayle hasn't picked up on it and I haven't said anything about it."
CJ: "Is there a problem in the notes that relates to her reluctance to walk with her sticks?"
Karen: "No, nothing identified."
CJ: "Do you think there should be?"
Karen: "Yes."

Commentary

Karen knew Mrs Kitchen primarily in terms of her operation and mobility. She did not know her in terms of the meaning the accident had for her and her fears for the future. As a consequence, Karen and others had tuned into Mrs Kitchen at the physical level rather than the emotional/psychological level.

Karen confronted Mrs Kitchen's reluctance to mobilise with her walking sticks. Karen was pleased with her response because she achieved the desired outcome without the anticipated conflict. However, she responded from her perception of what Mrs Kitchen *should* be doing, rather than understanding why Mrs Kitchen had been reluctant to use the sticks. Mrs Kitchen will never effectively use her sticks if she is afraid. As such, a cathartic/catalytic intervention may have been more appropriate than confrontation at this stage.

Karen felt uncertain about using confrontation and cathartic responses, supporting Burnard & Morrison's findings. She was motivated to avoid confrontation because she didn't want to upset the patient or feel uncomfortable, equating confrontation with conflict. Karen's actions reflected a cultural norm where patients were not involved in negotiating care and where decisions were made by nurses and doctors 'in the patient's best interests'. Within this culture Mrs Kitchen was at risk of being labelled 'difficult' or 'unco-operative' because she resisted using the prescribed sticks.

In her next session Karen said: "I followed up Mrs Kitchen. I asked her if she had a fear of using her sticks. She said she did have fear of falling again and then I couldn't take it any further."
CJ: "So what happened?"
Karen: "I asked her 'What are you going to do to regain your independence?' She said 'I have to do it'. I then offered to walk with her there and then, but I didn't seem to help her with her confidence at all."
CJ: "She's not here now?"
Karen: "She went home last Saturday with her zimmer frame. It would be

easier to use her sticks at home. The floor is not slippery as it is here and walls are nearer to hold onto if she did fall."

CJ: "Is this just her rationalising this?"

Karen: "Yes, I can understand the slippery floors though."

CJ: "What feelings are you left with?"

Karen: "Disappointed that she didn't get to use her sticks independently or for her to progress further in using her sticks with support."

CJ: "Could it have been different on reflection?"

Karen: "I don't think so. I can still carry it on – she's coming into the day unit on Thursdays. That eases the disappointment a bit."

CJ: "How did you feel when you asked her about her fear?"

Karen: "Expected a deeper, more meaningful conversation – I didn't get it."

CJ: "You could have got her to reflect on – 'I did have a fear'."

Karen: "Yes, but I couldn't see how to take it further."

CJ: "Can you see now?"

Karen: "No, I still can't."

CJ: "You go to the root of the problem, that it was psychological rather than physical."

Karen: "Yeah, I got to that."

We explored further the way Karen could have used cathartic and catalytic responses to help Mrs Kitchen talk through her fears.

CJ: "Using 'distraction' may also be a useful response; for example, saying to Mrs Kitchen 'Tell me about your life/house in London', whilst helping her to walk. This might be difficult because she will not want to be distracted. If so, just reflect that 'I don't want you to focus on walking!' Have you considered using relaxation tapes to help her relax?"

Karen: "There are a couple of ladies downstairs who might benefit. One lady already uses relaxation tapes to help her relax with her arthritic pain. She now lets the other lady use it."

CJ: "Also with arthritic pain?"

Karen: "No, compression pain. She gets very uptight about it. She was initially reluctant to use the tapes – 'I wouldn't dabble in any mystical stuff'."

CJ: "It worked?"

Karen: "It sent her to sleep!"

CJ: "Did you use a pain chart to monitor this?"

Karen: "She doesn't have any pain – she's just uncomfortable with it. It would be an interesting trial to use; we could get the other woman to use a pain chart."

I informed Karen of the relaxation tapes in the hospital.

Commentary

Karen had used her 'new' responses effectively with Mrs Kitchen. This was important 'trial and error' learning. Barriers to using these responses lay within her own lack of imagination, fear of competence, lack of knowledge, lack of belief in herself as a therapeutic tool. Yet Karen still saw herself as failing to 'fix it' for Mrs Kitchen, rather than seeing the response as the patient's responsibility. As a consequence, she remained anxious about Mrs Kitchen using her sticks, although she now saw the 'problem' differently.

Guided reflection was helping Karen shift from a 'fix it' mentality (essentially a mindset of doing for the patient and accepting responsibility for outcome) to working with the patient. The shift is characterised by an increased emphasis on using facilitative responses rather than authoritative responses (Box 5.2) and a creative autonomy to explore new ways of responding, such as distraction and relaxation.

'Being there' and touch

Karen's story suggested that many nurses feel they need to be doing something to fix the problem. Alison's story reflects that simply 'being there' and responding intuitively with touch is, in itself, a powerful therapeutic response that nurses underestimate.

REFLECTIVE EXEMPLAR 5.2: ALISON'S STORY

Alison is a senior staff nurse who shared an experience in group guided reflection about her feelings of uselessness and panic when accompanying a woman from ITU for a scan. The team was rushing her back to the ward. Alison noted that all she could do was to stroke the woman's hair whilst in the lift.

When she shared this experience, she was challenged by Nina, her guide and colleague, to reflect on that action. Alison felt she had done it intuitively, a reflection of her concern for this woman who was the same age as her, just 32. They returned to ITU where mechanical ventilation was recommenced. The woman's oxygen saturation recovered and she eventually made a full recovery.

Nina wrote:

"I could see that Alison had felt useless and helpless, that she felt she had no role in that lift. All she had managed to do was stroke Jane's hair. I felt it was important that she should be able to see that *being there* was her role. Nursing is said to be one of the few medical/healing professions that carries out a major portion of its functions through touch.

Alison was stroking Jane's hair as a means of reassurance, to imply a presence and to convey her sense of caring. Touch has the unique ability to communicate empathy without using words, words that Alison felt difficult and inappropriate to say in the confines of the lift. Additionally, it is suggested that when a patient is intensely stressed no other form of communication compares with the speed of response to the comforting effects of touch. In our notes of the supervision session we questioned whether touch could have an impact that would reduce anxiety and lead to improved blood pressure and oxygen saturation. The research subsequently reviewed cannot prove this quantifiably in the intensive care setting, but all the papers examined did indicate this probability.

Alison can feel reassured that her use of touch at this time in Jane's life, when she was critically ill and unconscious, was an attempt to communicate through one of the senses likely to be intact. When Alison instinctively reached out to stroke Jane's hair, she gave her support, she attempted to calm her, to ease her anxiety; she tried to ensure awareness of a caring presence and to communicate that Alison was *there for her*. Surely this was a most appropriate, fundamental and worthy role in the circumstances."

Commentary

Without doubt touch is a powerful response, as illustrated within Alison's story. Yet often touch is taken for granted. Consider your own use of touch. Are you aware when you touch your patients? Do you use touch in a deliberate or instinctive way? What impact does touch have on your patients or their families? What impact does touch have on you? Do you touch to convey your own feelings? What can you learn by reading and relating to Alison's story?

REFLECTIVE EXEMPLAR 5.3: JANET AND MICHELLE'S STORY

Consider Michelle's response to Mrs Denver, a woman admitted for a breast biopsy. Michelle is a staff nurse who has been qualified for 12 months. Janet is the ward sister. Janet had been working with me in guided reflection over two years and was implementing the Burford NDU model within the busy five-day surgical unit. The most significant change in practice for the nurses had been recognising the person rather than the disease-labelled patient; for example, understanding and responding to the meaning that having a breast lump and breast cancer meant for the woman.

Michelle: "She was a nurse, a pleasant lady. Next morning I was on an early doing the drugs. I asked her whether there was anything she needed. She said 'No ... oh I do feel a bit weepy' and she burst into tears. I pulled the drug trolley over and pulled the curtains around the bed. She said her friends had been saying how scared they would be if it was them ... she hadn't appreciated these feelings until now. She said 'Oh my husband and my children!' It made me think ... she's a nurse and she's so vulnerable. I don't know if I did any good."

Janet: "Put yourself in her shoes ... you spent half an hour with her. How would you have felt if a nurse did this for you? Nurses often underestimate the work they do with patients. Could you have done more?"

Michelle: "I made a conscious decision to blow the pills, no-one will come to any harm. It made me feel so vulnerable – what do you say?"

Janet: "Did you have to say anything? Nurses aren't very good at sitting and listening ... it's okay giving out information and advice.' "

Michelle: "The silence is difficult ... it's keeping quiet I find the hardest. Did we give her the opportunity to chat? Did we keep away because she was a nurse? Are we frightened of being patronising ... should she be treated any differently?"

Janet: "You are this patient's named nurse and therefore it was appropriate for you to spend time with her. Finding someone to take over the drugs or even finding the named nurse, if you hadn't been the named nurse, would have lost the spontaneous moment for this lady. Did you discuss this with other staff?"

Michelle: "Yes – we are not as sensitive to these ladies with breast lumps as we could be. Would a counselling course help? I'm at a loss to know what to say to them, am I helping or hindering? It's such a sensitive issue. They look jolly and jovial outside but inside it's like a bombshell!"

Janet: "Did you use touch?"

Michelle: "I put my hand on her arm when she apologised for crying. Not knowing her well enough stopped me holding her hand."

Janet: "Could you have done anything differently?"

Michelle: "I could have been more available to her preoperatively. I couldn't make it better for her ... change what was wrong."

Janet: "What would have happened if this had been a busier morning?"

Michelle: "I wouldn't have left her but I wouldn't have been so calm. I'd have been thinking about other work: premeds, eyedrops, and things ... thinking I wish you'd hurry up. That's really wrong – how do we get over that?"

Janet: "I don't really know. Perhaps as practitioners we need to be more prepared to defend our actions."

Commentary

Use ethical mapping to consider whether Michelle's decision to stop the drug round and respond to Mrs Denver was the right decision. Perhaps Michelle did not prioritise her work enough to react to Mrs Denver's distress within the moment. She could acknowledge her uncertainty in knowing and managing her priorities. In choosing to be with Mrs Denver, Michelle chose not to be with other patients. Yet Michelle must be able to justify her decision, to confront others' perceptions of priorities when these are misplaced and resist any blame as a consequence. The most significant caring factor was Michelle's availability to Mrs Denver at that moment. Although Michelle knew she could not fix it for Mrs Denver, she felt that pressure as she absorbed Mrs Denver's distress.

The drug round reflects a task approach to nursing – all patients receive medication at uniform times, helped by the routinisation of drug administration times into fixed patterns. The task is an efficient way of ensuring people get their medication. However, because the administration of drugs is routinised it may detract from seeing and responding to the individual's needs. Tasks also break up the pattern of holistic care by fragmenting aspects of the whole. The counter argument is that the practitioner does a mini drug round just for her patients. Giving someone a drug is a moment for reflection to consider the efficacy of the various drugs, to teach, to be with the patient. Unfortunately, the attitude is often just to get the task done. The task becomes a routine to structure the day.

At Burford we deconstructed the drug round. Each primary or associate nurse was responsible for ensuring their own patients received their drugs. Yet Burford had only nine beds, far removed from a 30-bed surgical ward.

Reflect on the routines and tasks of your day and consider whom they benefit. In a world of shrinking resources, practitioners are at great risk of role overload that inevitably squeezes the caring aspect and heightens the dilemma of managing priorities. Betz & O'Connell (1987) describe role overload as being responsible for more tasks than an individual could perform within shift time. They note that role overload is greater when associated with perceived 'low-level' tasks and more paperwork. As Leslie noted: 'When I focus on patient care my stress goes down and when I focus on workload, interviews, case conferences my stress goes up" (Johns, 1998a).

One response to shrinking resources is to break down the 'shift-bound' culture and move to a new culture of carrying out role responsibility. When practitioners felt valued, they felt they had a choice about issues and felt in control of their use of time. Otherwise they resisted and resented intrusion on personal time (Johns, 1998a). This understanding is significant in creating a culture of responsibility and support. The two must be in balance. However, such a culture is always open to abuse by unscrupulous organisations who see nursing as a prime target for resource savings.

Managing priorities

The pressure of workload emerged as a significant factor in Michelle's availability to Mrs Denver. Certain pressures, for example work overload, appear to accentuate the effects of other pressures (Marshall, 1980). Within a busy world of finite resources, the effective practitioner understands and balances competing priorities. The use of time always presents an ethical dilemma. 'Do I spend time with this person or with that person?' 'Who has the greater need?' 'How do I determine this?' Within hospitals, the organisation is geared towards tasks based on hierarchical prioritising. Box 5.3 sets out a hierarchy of priorities that existed within the culture of a community hospital that was attempting to implement primary nursing (Johns, 1989).

Box 5.3   Work priorities hierarchy.

> *First priority* – Executing medical responses and physical care
>
> *Second priority* – Complying with organisational demands, for example in completing documentation
>
> *Third priority* – Talking with patients

When I fed this understanding back to the hospital's practitioners, they were uncomfortable because it shattered the illusion that they were practising holistic-based nursing. Yet so deep was this task approach to work that it could not easily be shrugged aside. Failure to comply with this hierarchy of priorities led to conflict within the team and with more powerful others whose interests were represented within the hierarchy. The solution was not to rearrange the hierarchy but to collapse it within a new culture of professional judgement and responsibility based on the unit's philosophy and the ability to make good judgements about priorities and negotiate care within the limits of possibility. Creating and sustaining an environment that supports caring practice is discussed in depth in Chapter 8.

Chapter 6

Knowing and Managing Self within Caring Relationships

Introduction

The stories shared have illuminated the significance of reflective writing to access and know caring. They also illuminate reflective writing as a therapeutic activity for the practitioner to sensitise self to the nuances of everyday practice, as a way to explore and find meaning in practice and life itself. The practitioner is not neutral. She 'sees' and responds to the person through a filter of her own concerns which need to be acknowledged, understood and ultimately managed so that they do not interfere with the way the practitioner perceives and responds to the needs of the patient and family.

REFLECTIVE EXEMPLAR 6.1: SIMON'S STORY

Consider the story Simon wrote about his caring for Bill and his family. Simon is a charge nurse on a medical ward. His story is a search for meaning in the suffering and joy he experienced, reflecting the deeply emotional aspect of holistic practice and the fundamental need to know and manage self. Simon wrote:

> "Nursing is a demanding profession. The commitment we invest in our roles provides us with our greatest source of reward – the ability to use our position to aid others. This interpersonal aspect of nursing when encountering people at their most vulnerable is the foundation of our practice and its fulfilment the foundation of our satisfaction even though the price of constant exposure to emotionally challenging situations can be very high. Can we avoid this expense? Or can we grow as nurses and as people through it? Can we become overexposed to death and dying, resulting in emotional detachment that undermines holistic care and prevents us from using ourselves in therapeutic ways or learning from the experience?
>
> By reflecting on my involvement with Bill, a 40-year-old man who died

of cancer, I am attempting to discover the factors that influenced my feelings and actions. Standing at a shade over six feet tall, weighing a muscular 14 stone, the smiling face on the photograph provided a shocking contrast to the image of its owner sleeping in the bed. I use the word 'shocking' in response to how cancer specialises in the distortion of features and expression more rapidly than a cosmetic surgeon's knife and in a fashion that only first-hand witnesses could believe. When the bones, normally concealed beneath a physique developed through good living and exercise, become not only visible but the dominating feature in Bill's appearance, it becomes cruel irony of nature that many years of development can be so undone at a rate that growth can never equal.

We described Bill as being cachexic, a single word to describe so much. As professionals we are very comfortable and familiar with our terminology. It becomes very easy to use and the words can soften the impact of their meaning. This is a user-friendly language that cannot begin to portray what it describes. Cachexia is defined as abnormally low weight, weakness and general bodily decline associated with chronic disease, most notably cancer.

In reality, however, it is the image that Jane [Bill's wife] tries to spare her sons – Joe and Tim – from seeing, fearing nightmares and difficult 'why?' questions. It is the sight of a loving son, a devoted husband and doting father reduced to a living skeleton barely able to acknowledge everything in life that is dear to him and those who love him struggling with their pain.

Bill was admitted to our ward when symptoms of his lung cancer began to overwhelm him and his family. It had been a short disease process typical in its presentation and diagnosis. The dry cough that had failed to respond to linctus annoyed Jane so much that she wore down Bill's reluctance and persuaded him to go to the GP who sent Bill for a chest X-ray. The film showed a shadow that in turn resulted in bronchoscopic biopsy and diagnosis. Simple, systematic and effective intervention. It is the impact that has the medical profession floundering like a bully having its bluff called; 'So what are you going to do now?'. You can almost sense the taunt.

Radiotherapy was marginally successful in reducing the size of the shadow. Isn't 'shadow' an easy word to use, avoiding the dreaded 'c' word but managing to remain mysterious, sinister and often, for the patient, ambiguous? But tragically, its postponement of the inevitable was its only consequence. Subsequent community management with the input of Macmillan nurses had kept Bill at home until uncontrollable pain and nausea necessitated admission to hospital. The original plan was to achieve symptom control to facilitate discharge as soon as possible. However, the best laid plans of mice and men . . .

Bill was nursed on a pressure-reducing mattress in response to his elevated Waterlow score caused by his weight loss and poor appetite. An intravenous infusion was commenced to correct dehydration and a sub-cutaneous infusion pump containing diamorphine and cyclizine. The dosage was calculated on the basis of the previous inadequate dose and was devised to achieve instant pain control. The cyclizine was initiated to alleviate his nausea. It was decided that initial symptom control would be followed by a fuller assessment of Bill's needs. Bill had lost his appetite and was unable to keep fluids down long enough for them to be of any value. He looked dry and blood tests confirmed this impression. Secondary to this reduced fluid intake, Bill experienced oral candida and some painful oral ulcers. Bill could feel the pain through his chest wall and assessment using a 'pain ruler' confirmed its severity. Antifungal and ulcer medications were prescribed for Bill's mouth and regular oral care was provided. The dia-morphine and cyclizine were initially effective but the diamorphine needed to be increased within hours to achieve maximum pain control.

Bill's condition stabilised over the next couple of days. The nausea and pain were well controlled. He tolerated oral fluids and fluid-based sup-plements well and his stomatitis improved. Bill's condition improved enough for him to have visits from his sons. They were aged eight and 12 years old. Jane had protected them as much as possible by shielding them from seeing their father when he had been feeling particularly ill and looking unwell. During this period, over 3–4 shifts, I got to know Bill quite well. He was intelligent, articulate and we shared mutual interests in sport and music. I would sit with him and debate areas of mutual interest. We shared a similar sense of humour and managed to make each other laugh frequently. I wished I had the opportunity to know Bill for longer.

Bill and I were disagreeing about England's World Cup chances as I left the ward for two days off. Bill invited me to call round and see him when he was at home as we were aiming for discharge in the next two days. I replied that I would try but I knew deep down that I wouldn't. Not because I doubted that Bill would get home, but once a patient goes home we prepare for the next one. Our busy schedules are exactly that and how much time and involvement can we invest?

On one occasion, whilst completing some paperwork, I found myself watching Bill as his family visited. The indelible image was that of seeing the boys sit at the foot of the bed and almost simultaneously touch their dad's feet as their mum hugged him. The boys so needed the physical contact but seemed so reserved and hesitant until Bill held out his arms and the boys rushed to him and held him as tightly as they could. They seemed scared to let go and Bill, eyes closed, tried to absorb and retain every precious moment knowing how valuable this time was. Later that evening, I checked on my sleeping son and cried as I recalled what I had seen earlier. My emotions were a combination of anger at how people's lives are so senselessly destroyed and fear generated where the fine line between life and death is made so visible and where our own mortality is questioned.

Returning from my days off, I viewed the patient information board and noted that Bill had been transferred into the sideroom. I immediately asked the nurse looking after Bill what had happened. She informed me that Bill was very ill and close to death. Bill had become increasingly dyspnoeic due to the development of an extensive pleural effusion. A pleural aspiration had been performed which alleviated some of his breathlessness. However, the effusion was a sign of general deterioration that warranted increased analgesia and a sedative to control his developing agitation.

Bill's deterioration was rapid, the disease's only concession to Jane's feelings. 'He's not in pain, is he?' Jane enquired urgently. Before I could respond, Jane continued, 'I wish we could have got him home'. I answered Jane, describing that Bill was asleep and peaceful, indicating that the medication was being effective and that we were continually assessing his condition. Jane was obviously feeling some distress that Bill had not got home as she repeated her statement to herself shaking her head and crying.

'I think Bill's main concern was to have you all here,' I responded, looking towards the sons, trying to highlight to them how important their presence was to their dad. 'Holding his hand and talking to him is the most you can do regardless of where you are,' I continued. Jane forced a smile in my direction and nodded in agreement. She turned her attention to Bill and her sons. Feeling somewhat uncomfortable with the ensuing silence, I asked a typically English question, 'Can I get you a cup of tea or anything?'.

Bill's family visited at regular intervals as he slipped into unconsciousness. I continued to assess the effectiveness of our clinical care and let the family know that I was there for them should they need anything. Within an hour Bill died. I stood silently, deprived of the sanctuary of offering tea. I withdrew to allow the family privacy. Jane was very protective of her sons and through her grief she remained strong for them. They were distraught and through their tears their eyes betrayed a vacant, disbelieving look; in this instant they were experiencing emotions with demands beyond their tender years. Their sobbing provided a heartbreaking image and I was revisited by the twin impostors of anger and fear and a feeling of frustration at my helplessness.

I offered my condolence simply by expressing how sorry I was and instinctively touched Tim's arm as he stood next to me. Jane took my hand and thanked me for all I had done. I repeated how sorry I was and said how I liked Bill a lot. She seemed to appreciate this and smiled. I was glad that I had told Jane this. I felt for some reason that this was important to me as I knew that I would not get another chance to hint at the impact looking after Bill was having on me. The practical aspects were discussed with Bill's brother-in-law and provided almost a sense of relief that comes with taking refuge in practices over which we have some control.

Bill required a subtle balance of physical and psychological care typical in palliative nursing. But its influence on me as a person, and subsequently as a nurse, was atypical. I found myself experiencing fear, helplessness, inadequacy, anger and levels of distress that I had not felt since my earliest nursing exposure to death and dying. Farrar (1992) recognised these emotions in novices. However, my experience is far beyond novice so why do I seem to be regressing? I initially perceived these feelings to be barriers to effective care as they can elevate stress levels and compromise my ability to carry out clinical care objectively. In providing psychological support I have always felt it prudent to keep some distance between my empathy and my personal feelings, a kind of conditional empathy whose presence is determined by my feelings of discomfort and my emotional self-defence. In short, the experience has exposed barriers in my attitudes that, unless resolved, will impact negatively upon practice.

My reflection illuminates the darkest area of my practice and discovers the source of my fear, anger and frustration and guides me in my attempts to learn from them and apply my understandings in practice. Bill and I had much in common which stimulated me to empathise to the extent that I was forced to confront my own personal experiences of loss and my own mortality. I felt helpless at not being able to alter the course of Bill's prognosis or lessen the impact on his wife and sons. These are perfectly normal human responses but need to be fully understood to turn them into positive emotions, rather than areas for personal conflict and distress. The majority of my nursing practice has been in a care of the elderly environment and my dealings with palliative care in my age group have been very limited. In managing the needs of older patients, I can see that I could more easily employ my coping mechanisms that dilute the personal impact and subsequently the felt distress.

This is not to say that terminal disease is any less tragic for the people involved or that it requires any less skill or commitment on the nurses' behalf. But I am able to rationalise the event and see it more objectively. In examining my thoughts related to my own mortality, it is clear to me that it is a subject that I have actively avoided. McSherry (1996) details the importance of discovering our attitudes to mortality to resolve our barriers to death and dying. The experience of observing the trauma of Bill's sons brings back memories of my own father's death that I have not allowed to impact on my nursing due to the upset that they still evoke. Reisseter & Thomas (1986) state that these are the very emotions that we need to expose and incorporate into our practice. In avoiding applying my own experience actively in my practice, I am denying a major source of personal knowing. Utilising this knowing would enhance my care as I could use my subsequent increased capacity for empathy to understand my patients' needs more acutely and view this closeness as a bridge rather than a barrier.

Applying my own anxiety and fear of death and dying to provide a door to another's actions and thoughts rather than a subject to be dispelled immediately on appearance gives me the opportunity to provide true holistic care. The question 'How would I feel if that were me?' should not only be accepted but encouraged if holism is our objective. In revisiting my father's illness, I am reminded of the doctors, nurses and therapists that we came into contact with and the way they made me feel. Whispering at the foot of the bed, head shaking when reading the notes and being stared at by curious student nurses are memories that I seldom, if ever, relate to my own ideas of nursing. Do I whisper over my patients, leave patients perplexed and terrified with the shake of my head or the raising of an eyebrow or forget the individual right not to be a source of medical curiosity? I wish that I could cast the first stone at these sins but in reality I fear that I cannot. I worry that a lack of true empathy that can prevail when we lessen our humanness leads to a provision of care guided by a form of nursing 'autopilot' that demands little from us. I am equally reminded of the staff who respected my father and our family with their time, skills and most of all their understanding that meant so much to us so much of the time.

I want to leave a positive impression of my caring on those with whom I come into contact and recognise and resist the factors that reduce this possibility. I hope that Jane's memories of Bill's hospital care are reassuring. I will then have achieved something. At times I feel like a voyeur, impotent, unable to achieve practical goals that would make myself or Bill's family feel better. The danger of containing these feelings is that I carry them around with me into the next similar scenario, immediately creating a barrier.

Through reflection I am now in a better shape to use my frustration and anger to enhance my care. Being able to value the care I give reduces my frustration and allows me to accept my limitations, whilst my anger can be channelled into striving to improve in all areas of practice. Anger experienced by patients and their families is often inevitable as part of the grieving process (Kübler-Ross, 1969), but its impact can be damaging as there is no justifiable recipient to direct it at. In harnessing memories of my own anger when coping with my father's illness, I can detect this in difficult or aggressive people and avoid dismissing them as irritating or their behaviour as meaningless.

The anger I felt at seeing a man deprived of the opportunity to love his sons, enjoy and nurture their growth has to be managed and resolved to avoid extreme levels of stress and potential burn-out. In response to this, I am committed to working with our Macmillan team to establish a support network for nurses on the ward to explore, share and hopefully resolve emotional fall-out from the personal impact of our work. I am now a more complete nurse through knowing Bill. If experience is expensive it is also enlightening, supportive and rewarding.

Possibility and vulnerability of the therapeutic use of self

Simon's story draws attention to the significance of the practitioner knowing and managing self to be available to work with the patient and family. The possibility and vulnerability of the therapeutic use of self is evident in Simon's response to Bill and his family's needs. Care of the dying is comprehensively documented as being difficult and stressful (Hingley & Cooper, 1986; Bailey & Clarke, 1989), and remains an area surrounded by fears and anxiety within both society and nursing (Field, 1989).

A study by Reisseter & Thomas, (1986) showed a significant relationship between high-quality palliative care, reduced stress levels and an individual nurse's ability to draw on personal experience of death and dying. This would seem to indicate that nurses who have the motivation and ability to reflect upon their experience as a method of development are better equipped to respond effectively to the needs of their patients. In contrast, Atkinson *et al.* (1990) detail the way people deal with personal loss by viewing it in abstract terms that 'prevent us from internalising and personalising questions surrounding our mortality or death.' The research indicates that nurses who are able to utilise their own experience to enhance their personal knowledge are in a better position to manage the need of their patients and the impact upon themselves and to explore further the issues involved. Through reflection, we can harness this personal knowledge. In doing so, we can reveal and understand the feelings, attitudes and prejudices that guide our behaviour that Hall (1964) has claimed is essential to our development.

The x-ray film showed a shadow, the shadow of death that hovered within Bill and over his family. How do we learn to live in the shadow of death with its distress and suffering? Simon felt this suffering and suffered himself. Rinpoche (1992) observes:

> 'Suffering ... gives you such an opportunity of working through and transforming it. The times you are suffering can be those when you are most open, and where you are extremely vulnerable can be where your greatest strength really lies. Say to yourself then: "I am not going to run away from this suffering. I want to use it in the best and richest way I can, so that I can become more compassionate and more helpful to others". So whatever you do, don't shut off your pain; accept your pain and remain vulnerable. And don't we know only too well, that protection from pain doesn't work, and that when we try to defend ourselves from suffering, we only suffer more and don't learn what we can from the experience?' (p. 316)

Simon used the model for structured reflection (Box 3.5) when he commenced reflection. Now, a year later, he weaves the cues together as a whole story, yet the cues can be discerned within the whole. The reflective cues (Box 2.2) 'How do I feel about this person?' and 'How is this person feeling?' are particularly significant for Simon to consider himself inter-subjectively as therapeutic. The focus for his reflection was his strong feelings. His effort was to make sense of these, not to rationalise them but to learn through them, to manage them without diminishing them, because his feelings are central to his own being and the care he gives.

By this I do not mean the practitioner somehow 'brackets' his feelings, attitudes, concerns, etc. in order to become detached from himself because in such circumstances, there would be nothing of himself to give! Yet the stereotype of the *professional* nurse as being detached prevails. To respond from a holistic perspective to the patient or family, the practitioner needs to engage with his feelings, often feelings of anxiety, distress and suffering, any negative feelings towards him or any preoccupation that might interfere with the ability to recognise and respond to the patient's concerns. Negative feelings tie up energy that is no longer available for therapeutic work.

Involvement

To respond to the other in their humanness and their suffering requires an involvement in which the consequences cannot be known although they can usually be intuited. In this sense, it is an unconditional willingness to become involved. However, there is a danger of overinvolvement when the therapeutic vision becomes blurred through entanglement with the other (Morse, 1991). This is always a risk when practitioners do not know themselves or have not been prepared to use the therapeutic self.

As noted above, practitioners often describe a fear of 'getting in too deep' , yet the dialogue with the other and dialogue with self makes it possible to be open and authentic, necessary for 'working with' relationships and exploring the depths together. The practitioner does not set out to 'fix it' for the other but to work with the other to help them find meaning in the experience. As the stories show, being faced with another's distress and suffering is not comfortable. Within a trusting relationship it becomes possible to express uncertainty and distress. Caring is reciprocated – the patient or relative cares for the nurse because they are cared for. This reciprocation is inevitable and must be expected and accepted because in being cared for, the other has a need to give something back.

The effective practitioner learns to tune into the patient or family member to gauge the appropriate level of involvement at that moment. By reading the patient's pattern, the patient's desire for involvement can be appreciated and negotiated within the ongoing dialogue. Where resistance is felt, either because the patient or relative demands an inappropriate level of involvement or because the practitioner for whatever reason resists involvement, then the practitioner reflects and responds appropriately. From this perspective, all nurse–patient/family relationships can be viewed along a continuum of resistance and reciprocation (Johns, 1999b). Resistance and reciprocation, like concern and vulnerability, are two sides of the same coin. The relationship will ebb and flow within the unfolding rhythm of the caring dance. It is a deeply focused intimacy. Simon's story illustrated the way a relationship can be fraught when the practitioner has not learnt to manage self within such relationships. Wrapped up in their own concerns, the practitioner may impose expectations on the patient or resist the demands put upon them, with loss of synchronicity.

The nature of nurse–patient relationships

The work of Morse (1991), Ramos (1992), May (1991) and Fossbinder (1994) offers insight into the nature of the nurse–patient relationship (Johns, 1999b). The resistance–reciprocation dialectic was developed through assimilating and transcending Morse's (1991) unilateral-mutual nurse–patient relationship types dichotomy (Box 6.1). Morse constructed her 'types' in an effort to make sense of the outcome of nurse–patient relationships rather than knowing the practitioner's intent. From a holistic perspective the practitioner would always intend to establish a connected relationship. This holds true even if the time span for connection is very brief. In other words, the connection intent is a state of mind.

Box 6.1 Typology of nurse–patient relationships (Morse, 1991).

Unilateral – The nurse or the patient resists the level of involvement demanded from the other → breakdown.

Mutual – The nurse and patient agree an accepted level of reciprocity. There are four types:
   (1) clinical: The nurse views the person primarily as a patient with a medical label, usually within a brief time span.
   (2) therapeutic: As clinical but over a longer time span where the nurse primarily views the patient within a clinical label yet also acknowledges the person to establish trust.
   (3) connected: The nurse primarily views the patient as a person and the patient's concerns are primary.
   (4) overinvolved: Characterised as an intimate relationship in which the nurse's perception has become blurred as a consequence of emotional involvement.

If you are admitted to my unit or I visit you for the first time in the community, I ask myself (using the Burford reflective cues) 'Who is this person?' 'What meaning does this health event have for this person?' 'How is this person feeling?' I have no intention to establish a unilateral, clinical or therapeutic type relationship with you. To do so would be a contradiction and a focus for reflection to be resolved.

Ramos (1992) identified embodied impasses or resistance factors within the practitioner that limited their ability to realise connected types of relationships. The first impasse was emotional involvement that reflected the nurse's failure to draw boundaries between self and the other, reminiscent of Morse's overinvolvement type. The second impasse was the practitioner's need to control the patient's experience in order to protect the patient and to manage her own anxiety.

Consider your own level of involvement with particular patients. Do you tune into the appropriate balance of involvement? Who sets the level of involvement? Does the patient or family member reciprocate? Are you resisting the patient or family member? If so, what factors lead you to resist? Can you overcome this?

REFLECTIVE EXEMPLAR 6.2: HILDA

Even for experienced practitioners it is not always easy to monitor and manage self to remain available to the patient. Practitioners unwittingly get drawn into the patient's angst.

In one guided reflection session (Johns, 1993, 1998a), Jade, an experienced primary nurse, said:

> "Hilda told me I was horrid. I asked her why. She said it was because I had made her stand and take a few steps. I reminded Hilda that she had agreed this action with the primary nurse and her husband the previous day as recorded in the care plan. Her response to this was, 'I didn't agree to anything no matter what anyone said!'. Hilda implied that 'we enjoyed bullying her', which upset me. I told her that 'if we wanted things to be easy we would just leave you', which brought an almost predictable response from Hilda, 'Just leave me alone', which I then did. I felt pressured at this time with the needs of other patients. It made me feel uncomfortable all morning."
>
> *CJ*: "Could you have acted differently?"
>
> *Jade*: "No – it would be just the same. I had taken the right decision and made the right action based on the chat I had with the primary nurse yesterday."
>
> *CJ*: "You seem angry with Hilda."
>
> Jade recognised her caring dilemma: "We don't come to work dressed in a suit of armour to protect yourself from all this shit... you just feel you are a target for people to fire at." Jade noted that this experience had affected her relationship with Hilda: "I went back later to do her dressing and she just pulled away, didn't communicate, closed her eyes to dismiss me."

Commentary

Jade reflected on her dilemma of whether she should have made Hilda act contrary to her own wishes. Jade had to be certain that she was acting in

Hilda's best interests rather than her own wish to carry out planned care. Jade, as an associate nurse, should not blindly follow planned care. She needed to make a judgement as to whether the planned care was still appropriate for the patient's needs. Whether Hilda had agreed one thing yesterday was history. She may have merely complied yesterday and now, faced with the reality of this decision, she felt quite differently.

Jade noted that she continued to feel awful about this experience some days later, which she rationalised as oversensitivity. She was unable to avoid these awful feelings because of her concern. Hilda's rejection of her also made her feel angry. One way of dealing with such mixed feelings was to blame Hilda. However, Jade also felt bad for feeling angry with Hilda. It was as though she were on a merry-go-round of energy-sapping emotions towards herself and Hilda. Jade lived the dilemma of deciding what would be therapeutic for Hilda; on one hand, Hilda hated being in hospital and wanted to go home to be with her husband but on the other hand, she wanted to be left alone because she felt so tired. Hence Hilda was ambivalent about her rehabilitation and about her level of dependence on the nurses. Jade had not read this pattern. Jade's guilt reflected the way she perceived herself as failing to care. Dickson (1982) describes a 'compassion trap' whereby practitioners get trapped by their own concern or ethic of care, as if they have assumed all responsibility for the way the patient feels.

The consequence of the breakdown was failure to maintain an existential dialogue with Hilda. The confrontation led to a breakdown of connection because of a mutual need to control the situation in response to their respective anxieties. Noddings (1984) noted that the practitioner's sense of being overwhelmed, resulting in feelings of guilt and conflict, was the inescapable risk of caring. The balance between concern and being overwhelmed was a fine line for Jade to tread.

I asked Jade whether she had talked this over with her colleagues. She said she hadn't because she didn't want to burden them with her problems. In other words she limited her opportunity to take the armour off. The issue of effective support is discussed in Chapter 7. I mention it here to draw attention to the way Jade, like Leslie, had 'stewed in her juices' (Hall, 1964), unable to extricate herself from her entanglement with Hilda. The consequence was that Jade's ability to be available to work with Hilda was compromised.

From a guidance perspective I use a visualisation technique to enable practitioners such as Jade to put strong emotions into the 'space' between us so the emotions can be looked at for what they are and understood. Boundaries between self and other can be delineated and responsibility put into the perspective of holistic values. Guilt can be shredded. Afterwards the practitioner is usually successful in leaving some of the emotion behind in the 'space', having come to an understanding of herself and what she needs to do now or in future situations. Developing this sense of 'space' also nurtures reflection-within-the-moment, to help the practitioner recognise her emotional response and put into the space within the moment in order to reflect and respond appropriately.

REFLECTIVE EXEMPLAR 6.3: BASIL AND MRS ROBINSON

Resistance by the patient, relative or nurse can lead to the practitioner being less available to work with the patient, perhaps to the extent of creating an adversarial relationship.

Leslie shared the difficulty he had working with Mr Robinson's wife:

"Basil is 76, he was transferred to us two weeks ago for rehabilitation following a stroke some six weeks previously. He has quite a severe right-sided weakness. He is very heavy and has not made a lot of progress with physiotherapy. He is not very communicative, in fact more communicative with his wife than he is with us.

His wife decided he would be better off at home than here and therefore wanted him discharged as soon as possible. I said I could see her point of view but felt he should stay in hospital another 7–10 days for therapy. She said, 'No, I want him home'. I felt she wasn't listening any more to us so I arranged a discharge package and talked this through with the GP, who agreed the discharge arrangements and felt that the best thing to do was to go along with her wishes and pick up the pieces if we had to.

I felt that I had to put forward formal reasons for Basil to stay. In light of recent experiences with Tommy Hilton [complaint from the GP that discharge not planned well enough] and with Arun Eyles [complaint from district nurse that the discharge was inappropriate], I wanted the best possible care with agreement of all parties to minimise the risk of failure. Gayle [colleague] said it was defensive nursing."

CJ: "What was your reaction to that?"

Leslie: "I laughed about it and said perhaps it was. Gayle said she liked the letter I had written to the GP summarising the discharge."

CJ: "So the letter served two purposes. From a defensive point of view in light of criticism of recent other discharges, 'covering your back'. From a positive point of view it represented effective communication."

Leslie: "Yes, I felt the letter enabled me to establish effective communication with home care services although not necessarily with the family."

CJ: "Had you thought about sending Basil's wife a similar letter?"

Leslie: "No, I hadn't thought of that. When I tried to discuss the issues with her she always had a counter argument: physiotherapy – 'I know someone'; speech therapy – 'There is someone in the village'; how heavy he was – 'I've looked after people like him before'. I felt very frustrated at the time that the family weren't listening to me. I also had perverse feelings hoping that it would fail. I kept thinking the days after, 'When is it going to fail?'"

CJ: "Perhaps that's a natural reaction to not being listened to. You haven't been able to help her explore her feelings at all?"

Leslie: "No – she was a very bustly lady."

CJ: "Did you feel she would have shrugged you off if you had tried to explore the meaning of this [experience] for her?"

Leslie: "I did try but she did shrug me off."

CJ: "You felt unable to confront her with this?"

Leslie: "I could ring her up and suggest I visit to see how things are for her."

CJ: "That would certainly give them a strong message of caring for them. What about the district nurse?"

Leslie then identified and explored his options for further action: "I feel I did the best I could in the situation which felt 'distasteful', but I did manage a professional relationship even if I couldn't manage the 'personal' relationship I would have liked. From an accountability factor I did what was needed. I felt I was therapeutic without realising it."

CJ: "What does 'therapeutic' mean to you in this context?"

Leslie: "I tried to think of being therapeutic as resulting in feeling warm."

CJ: "You seem to need this warmth feedback from your relationships."

Leslie: "Yes, it makes it easier. It's problematic otherwise."

CJ: "To give a lot you need to take a lot?"

Leslie: "Yes. I need them to be grateful, but then why should I expect them to be?"

CJ: "You need to put that into perspective."

Leslie: "Yes. [laughs]"

When Leslie explored alternative ways of responding, he acknowledged his need to avoid confrontation with Mrs Robinson: 'I know I'm not good at confrontation.' At the end of the session I asked Leslie how he felt about Mrs Robinson now. Leslie: 'Puzzled really. A bit sorry that we didn't get through to each other but even though we didn't, I did my best in a professional sense".'

I suggested that Leslie should reflect on the nature of his relationship with Mrs Robinson within Robinson & Thorne's typology (Box 4.8). Leslie hoped that any relative's expectations, fears and needs would be identified and responded to appropriately. As such, Mrs Robinson's naive trusting that Leslie and other staff would share her needs would remain intact. This point highlights the essential need for a dialogue whereby expectations can be stated and negotiated within a climate of care. Clearly this level of relationship had not been achieved as Mrs Robinson had become very disenchanted. The relationship was stuck at this level because Leslie and Mrs Robinson were locked into a win–lose scenario that blocked the possibility of developing guarded alliance. There were no winners. Leslie felt stressed and guilty, Mrs Robinson was angry.

Commentary

The experience highlights the crucial significance of seeing and responding to the whole family in terms of the cue questions 'What support does this person have in life?' and 'How does the person view the future for themselves and others?'. Mrs Robinson felt peripheral to the caring situation when she needed to be central. Her disillusionment can be understood. She is herself in deep crisis as her normal life has disintegrated.

The failure to establish an effective existential dialogue led to breakdown and conflict, simply because Leslie could not tune into this woman's needs, notwithstanding how difficult she made this for him. It was as if Leslie had lost sight of Mrs Robinson and when he saw her again, he met a disillusioned woman. His interpretation of the situation was misplaced yet even on reflection, he could not see her perspective because he was entangled in the conflict. If conflict could have been surfaced and openly tackled, then it might have been resolved, leading to mutual benefit for patient, wife and nurse, even though this might have been uncomfortable.

Mrs Robinson resisted Leslie's desired level of involvement which led to mismatched expectations. When Mrs Robinson failed to reciprocate Leslie's concern, he simply gave way to her demands and withdrew emotionally from her, symbolised in his 'professional' rather than 'personal' involvement. Consequently, rather than working with her at this significant moment, Leslie found himself working against her. Yet she had real needs as manifested through her anxiety.

Leslie admitted to 'being no good at confrontation', indicating how he equated confrontation with conflict because he had failed to establish a relationship in which confrontation could be therapeutic rather than disintegrating into a 'win–lose' situation. Leslie needed to be challenged because he didn't know how much his need for personal or warm relationships interfered with achieving his 'professional role'. Leslie spoke as if the two roles are distinguishable and he moves from one, the professional role, into the personal role, whereas one is just the rationalisation for failing in the other.

At the end of the session, Leslie retorted that he was human too with human vulnerability and the right not to be abused by relatives. Of course, he is absolutely right yet his retort highlights the necessity to know and manage self if practitioners choose to work as nurses from a holistic perspective. He was only abused because he failed to read the situation adequately and respond appropriately. As a guide, my role is not to pass judgement of failure but to acknowledge that there is a real world and that it is tough at times. As such we must give ourselves a break and not judge ourselves too harshly.

REFLECTIVE EXEMPLAR 6.4: MAVIS AND JOY

Consider the way Karen establishes and maintains an appropriate level of involvement in her relationship with Mavis, a respite care patient, and Mavis's daughter Joy. Karen has been qualified for just six months. Note the way each session builds on the previous session, illustrating the way issues are anticipated, applying new understandings and actions, and subsequently reflected. Reflect on the supervision process, notably the balance of high challenge and high support and the way the reflective model cues (Box 2.2) are woven within the dialogue.

Session 13

Karen first talked about her relationship with Mavis and Joy in her 13th guided reflection session:

> "It's the first time I've seen Mavis as Joy describes her at home. For the last few months Joy has been saying how demanding she is at home – doesn't want Joy to go out. Joy feels trapped, it's affecting her marriage. I haven't seen that before when Mavis was here. I'm just observing how she is this time. She is much more demanding ... for example, take off my tights, put that there, etc."
> *CJ:* "What are your choices?"
> *Karen:* "To go along with it."
> *CJ:* "Do you have other choices?"
> *Karen:* "To challenge Mavis's behaviour; for example, to ask her for more politeness, to ask her why she is acting differently."
> *CJ:* "What are the consequences of 'going along with it'?"
> *Karen:* "She would receive care here as she gets at home."
> *CJ:* "Does her daughter do everything for her?"
> *Karen:* "Yes."
> *CJ:* "But very grudgingly?"
> *Karen:* "Yes. I think it's getting that way."
> *CJ:* "You're not sure?"
> *Karen:* "I'm not sure if 'grudgingly' is the right word. She's getting tired."
> *CJ:* "But she's complaining to you?"
> *Karen:* "She's justifying it; what Mavis did for her when she was a little girl."
> *CJ:* "Like repaying debts?"
> *Karen:* "Yes."
> *CJ:* "Caring from a sense of duty?"
> *Karen:* "Very much."
> *CJ:* "Are you doing something you don't want to do by mirroring Joy's behaviour with her mother at home?"

Karen: "It's not something you want to do. I'm carrying on for Joy's sake."

CJ: "You would like to change Mavis to make Joy's life easier; therefore, why do you 'carry on'?"

Karen: "Because it's the only way to observe the full picture at the moment."

CJ: "Let's look at your option to challenge Mavis."

Karen: "If I challenged her she might act differently than she does at home."

CJ: "Are you thinking that you might succeed in changing her behaviour here but not at home?"

Karen: "Yes. If I asked her to be polite when she's here, she would try desperately hard to be polite. Mavis is morally very correct. It would upset her too much. She would look at me with wide-eyed wonder and disbelief."

CJ: "Would we be asking her to be polite for our benefit rather than hers?"

Karen: "It wouldn't be for me – it would be for Joy's sake."

CJ: "What might be the reasons for her acting 'differently'? Could the reasons be organic – dementia?"

Karen: "I feel she is in a strop because Joy has gone on a holiday. She didn't want Joy to leave her."

CJ: "This has been happening for two years now. Do you think she has become more dependent? You could be cathartic to enable her to surface this anger – 'You seem angry that Joy has gone on holiday'."

Karen: "Thinking about the cathartic and catalytic way of acting [see Box 5.2], I don't think I often do that. That's why I probably chose the 'carry on as before' strategy. I have a fear of using these responses. I haven't used them before."

CJ: "A fear of the unknown? Fear of upsetting Mavis? Fear of cocking it up?"

Karen: "Yes, upsetting Mavis – being confrontational. Mavis has some environmental difficulties being here – a nosey woman in the same room and sharing a ward with a man as well."

CJ: "Are you suggesting that Mavis may be angry with us for these reasons? Consider the Burford model cue, 'What factors are significant in making this person's stay in hospital comfortable?'"

Karen: "I haven't considered whether these factors could have made her discontent..."

CJ: "Something else for you to consider. Do you feel you have a good relationship with Joy?"

Karen: "I feel she trusts me all of a sudden. I've always been open/friendly with her, I thought no more about it until I became her primary nurse. I don't know what else I need to do with her."

CJ: "Think about inviting her for a chat when she returns from her holiday, ostensibly to feed back how Mavis has been in hospital. How does that feel? How do you feel about Mavis?"

Karen: "I did think that she was a very nice lady. Now I'm beginning to think that she is more manipulative than I gave her credit for."

CJ: "Does that make you feel angry towards her?"

Karen: "Hesitant."

CJ: "It's important for you to understand how you feel about her because it may stop you from responding appropriately."

Karen: "That may be why I was going to observe."

CJ: "How do you feel about Joy?"

Karen: "I feel protective towards Joy, more protective for Joy than I do about Mavis."

CJ: "Are you at risk of being caught between two people?"

Karen: "Definitely – not knowing where my priorities lie."

Commentary

Karen's frustration with Mavis triggered her reflection. Karen illustrates the depth of knowing necessary to know the 'whole family' in order to respond to Joy and Mavis and to make sense of the conflicting and competing needs of each. However, Karen's sympathy lay with Joy, an emotional reaction rather than a deep understanding of the family's dynamics. As a consequence Karen felt entangled in a web of Joy's concerns to the extent that she began to re-evaluate Mavis as a 'nice person'.

Mavis was a private and proper person being compromised by her deteriorating intellect. Hence sharing a room with a man or with an intrusive other woman may well have been distressing for her, in context of her frustration at being left by her daughter/carer in hospital. Karen had not considered the impact of this environment on Mavis. The consequence was Karen's failure to tune into Mavis at this time, distracted by Joy's concerns and subsequently her own concerns.

Session 14

Karen: "I was so grateful we had the supervision session on it. I must make an appointment to see Joy soon as Mavis is coming in again in two weeks time."

CJ: "You are on a late today. Why not ring her this evening? This is called empowerment!"

Karen: "Maybe [cringes]. One of the reasons why I am so nervous is that I hoped other staff would have given me feedback about what I had written in the notes but I have received nothing. I was hoping we could rehearse how I'm going to put it to Joy."

CJ: "Okay – so you ring her."

Karen: "I could ask her to come here, although she will have to make an excuse to leave Mavis, or I could go and visit her in my own time, although Mavis would say, 'What's Karen doing here?'. It might be difficult to have a conversation without Mavis listening."

CJ: "In your own time?"

Karen: "I know ideally I should be able to do it in work time but the realities of trying to achieve this are difficult."

CJ: "Isn't it really just a question of looking at the off-duty and seeing where the overlaps are and being assertive? What's the best option?"

Karen: "To ask Joy to come here."

CJ: "What will you say to her on the phone?"

Karen: "I would explain the doubts I had about Mavis when she was in last and how she had different perceptions to those of Joy."

CJ: "How do you think she will react to this?"

Karen: "She's likely to panic – what's Mum been saying? What does Karen want to say to me?"

CJ: "Would you want to avoid that?"

Karen: "I would like not to panic her, but for her to see how important I see this is."

CJ: "Okay – let's rephrase this so you don't panic her."

Karen: "I could ask her if there is anything she would like to discuss about Mavis's admission beforehand."

CJ: "What if she says no? Or if she says the things over the phone?"

Karen: "I'm stuck."

CJ: "You may need a more direct invitation to her. For example, 'I've just returned from my holiday and I notice that Mavis is coming in. Can you pop in to see me at the hospital to have a chat about how things are at the moment and for me to give you feedback about how she was during her last stay?'. How does that feel?"

Karen: "Feels okay. If I went to her home it would become too social."

CJ: "So – she's here. What's your agenda?"

Karen: "I won't start by going straight in, some social chit chat first."

CJ: "For example, holidays?."

Karen: "Yes."

CJ: "Okay – start by relaxing the situation."

Karen: "No doubt the conversation will flow easily after that."

CJ: "Let's clarify your agenda – highlight how Mavis was last time and how she is now at home – then what?"

Karen: "Find out what she would like to happen – the reflective cue, 'How does she view the future for herself and others?'. Does she want Mavis to change or does she want my shoulder to lean on? What support does she have in life?"

CJ: "You might use a cathartic response – 'How is your husband feeling?'. Or if she expresses non-verbal distress – 'Joy, I can see this is upsetting you'. The aim would be to surface feelings because it *is* an emotional issue and feelings are important in making decisions. Do you feel able to deal with Joy's tears?"

Karen: "Yes."

CJ: "It will be useful to break down her pretences about keeping her mum at home."

Karen: "Yes. I need to determine what she really feels about keeping her mum at home, and then to look at ways to support her to do that."

We continued to explore these issues. At the end of the session Karen said she felt she could now act with some confidence.

Commentary

Karen was nervous and uncertain about how best to respond to Joy. She was anxious about messing it up or creating conflict. These concerns interfere with her being available to Joy and Mavis, constraining her involvement with this family. As a consequence Karen feels guilty because she knew she had failed to respond appropriately by avoiding the situation.

Session 15

Karen: "I didn't see Joy before she brought Mavis in. I was surprised that there were no grumbles from Joy. I said to her, 'Can I talk to you a minute without your mother hearing?'. I think I picked up on the fact that Joy was very relaxed and talking about everything under the sun except her mum! After all our rehearsing I just had to ask her outright. I was ready for a shock/horror reaction like I forecasted but I got none of it. She said, 'Yes, fine, when?' I think I was more amazed by that – more than she had been by my asking her to come in. I was trying to think of the reasons why there wasn't the shock/horror reaction. I thought either she trusts me totally or she saw it as an opportunity to have my whole attention or she wanted to talk to me too. But I don't think it was that because I didn't detect relief in her voice. I was glad I had asked her directly and hadn't pussy footed around trying to break it gently. I had been me."

CJ: "So somewhere you had felt pressure not to be yourself?"

Karen: "Yes. I feel that quite a lot down here anyway. I'm very conscious of north–south differences in nature because I have had bad reactions in the past to my directness and openness. Then I think I try to conform to how I think people are expecting me to behave down here. It seems that people act for a long time until they feel they've really got to know you."

CJ: "That sounds as if it interferes with communication?"

Karen: "Probably. I need to be on people's wavelength to be therapeutic."

CJ: "Even if that means conforming and compromising who you are to achieve this?"

Karen: "That's what I have been doing."

CJ: "The first five reflective cues of the Burford model enable you to get on the person's wavelength."

Karen: "After those five questions I understand their wavelength – it doesn't mean I'm with them on it."

CJ: "That's a good point. The skill is to monitor the impact of yourself on others and tune into their wavelength."

Karen: "I've realised I have been doing that more, being more direct and following things through."

CJ: "What's prompted that?"

Karen: "Thinking back to that meeting with Joy – she brought Wilf, her husband, along as well. That was fine. He was waffling on so much about something that I said, 'I'm asking you all these questions because I'm concerned about your marriage'."

CJ: "Do you think Wilf's waffling was avoiding issues?"

Karen: "No, that's Wilf. He's got to tell you everything about his life anyway."

CJ: "What was the impact of that, did their mouths drop open?"

Karen: "Not at all. They said, 'Thank you very much for telling us that, thank you for getting us here'. I wrote down in my diary 'direct questions get direct answers'."

CJ: "How did they respond?"

Karen: "They were initially quiet and then they started telling me things like, 'Why don't you tell Karen about the allowances. Oh yes, we can trust Karen with things like that'. It was as though I confirmed their hopes that I cared for them. Honesty was the biggest thing."

CJ: "How did that conversation end?"

Karen: "I reaffirmed to them that if they needed to talk to someone about their relationship with Mavis then they could talk to me – I was here. They responded to that by saying, 'If there's anything we can do for you in the world, anything, then please tell us and if we can help we will'. I definitely got across that I cared. They appreciated that. I wasn't sticking my nose in where it wasn't wanted."

CJ: "It beautifully illustrates the mutuality of caring."

Karen: "I wanted to say it went totally different to what I expected and it was good that I had that meeting to find out what they were planning in the future."

CJ: "What are they planning for the future?"

Karen: "They will have Mavis living with them until one or the other's health deteriorates or if Mavis's condition deteriorates to the point they feel incapable of caring."

CJ: "It's easier for them knowing you are with them now."

Commentary

By tuning into the other's wavelength and establishing an (existential) dialogue, mutuality of caring was established. Joy and Wilf were screaming out for someone to recognise them as people, as valid recipients of care. Karen did this. The situation had unfolded in ways we hadn't anticipated. Karen reacted intuitively, based on interpreting the situation. Karen's satisfaction is clear; she had liberated herself from previous norms that had limited her caring potential and realised herself as a caring person. Through reflection Karen could reaffirm her real self, legitimising and valuing her own qualities of being open and honest. Jourard (1971) noted:

> 'People learn to quash their real selves because they have learned to fear the consequences of authentic being and blind themselves to much of their real-self; impairing their ability to empathise with patients and disclose themselves.' (p. 184)

Jourard believes that such action leads to self-alienation, thus jeopardising the nurse's own health and limiting her ability to use herself in a therapeutic way. In enabling the growth of self, the self needs to be honoured and valued otherwise those with whom we work cannot be honoured and valued.

Session 20

It was not until session 20, four months later, that Karen picked up her work with Mavis and Joy.

Karen: "Mavis is very confused, very sad. Joy just says that Mavis is more confused and that she doesn't know what to do about it ... how to keep Mavis occupied. Mavis is less able to do her knitting, even to watch TV."
CJ: "And making more demands on Joy as a result?"
Karen: "Joy feels she should spend more time with her whilst in here."
CJ: "Can you reassure Joy about that?"
Karen: "I said that we should stimulate Mavis more while she is in hospital and pass on any good tips to Joy and Wilf for them to try out at home."
CJ: "Has anything emerged?"
Karen: "She can talk about the past with some understanding. Therefore old photographs, videos would be useful."

CJ drew Karen's attention to a book in the unit library that focused on reminiscence processes (Coleman, 1986).

CJ: "Joy would have to sit with her to accomplish that. Does she go to any clubs?"
Karen: "She says she won't go because she's deaf. Yet she'll sit with Ethel [another patient] and have a conversation. I really think she plays Joy up at

home, I really do. I'm toying with the idea of doing a home visit to clarify in my own mind if that is so."

CJ: "Even if she was, what could you do about it?"

Karen: "I'm not sure I could do anything, except be more empathic."

CJ: "What about other workers, for example the CPN for elderly?"

Karen: "No. The only contact is the GP. They have a lot of trust in him."

CJ: "Have you thought about using the CPN as a resource?"

Karen: "No, but that's a good idea. I haven't met her. This would be a good opportunity to do that."

CJ: "That leads you into ethical issues about individual needs versus resources."

Karen: "Knowing the home situation would lead to a better assessment. It would help Joy. For example, if Joy was helping Mavis to dress at home and Mavis was managing that by herself here, we could help Joy to change her management of Mavis at home."

CJ: "In that respect a complete reassessment might be quite useful. The CPN might help you with a cognitive assessment of time/place/space orientation, etc. However, you seem uncertain about a home visit."

Karen: "I feel claustrophobic about Joy and Wilf. I feel almost smothered by love with everything. I'm dodging them! So I'm reluctant to go and to feel even more closed in by them, stupid things like calling me 'sweetheart'."

CJ: "Yes. I can recall your aversion to being called endearing names by Elizabeth [patient]. You can't accept that from Joy and Wilf?"

Karen: "I have to be in a certain mood to accept it. I can appreciate this 'up here' but it's different when I'm 'down there'."

CJ: "It feels like a situation of 'involvement,' as if you want to take a step back and they want you to take a step forward."

Karen: "Yes, I'm maintaining a professional distance."

CJ: "Resisting them? It seems to be a recurring theme throughout your experiences – where to pitch your involvement with patients and families. Perhaps you want to take a step back because you don't know what's there?"

Karen: "Yeah, as if I don't know what demands it's going to make on me."

CJ: "Do you know the solution?"

Karen: "I know a solution: to do a home visit but to spell out the objectives and verbalise these to them – that this is *not* just a social visit but because..."

CJ: "In other words, set the boundaries for the visit and the relationship."

Karen: "Yes."

CJ: "I agree with your actions. It enables you to be positive rather than react negatively in resisting the need to 'step back' or resist them. It accepts their needs to be affectionate to you. You can monitor this and through setting objectives you can take control."

Karen: "Being in control – that's important. I can relate that to my earlier work with them. They make me feel like a big soft puppy."
CJ: "Do they have any children?"
Karen: "Joy has two children from a previous marriage."
CJ: "Relate this to your recurring theme of mothering and being mothered, as if you oscillate between these two roles in your relationships."

Commentary

Karen's involvement takes a paradoxical turn. Having worked hard to connect with Joy and Wilf, Karen recoils from the unexpected consequences. Joy and Wilf wish to reciprocate at an unacceptable level for Karen. Karen doesn't want to upset Joy and Wilf, yet resists this demand.

Karen struggled to deal with these feelings. In doing so, she withdrew from the family. Yet she also felt guilty about her resistance to these demands. As a result she felt entangled. She could not reciprocate the level of involvement demanded by the family. Yet neither could she resist it because of her concern for the family. She could not see that this was the way that Joy and Wilf expressed their care for her because she had became the rebellious child fighting against a level of intimacy that felt uncomfortable.

Session 21

Karen: "Mavis had agreed to go into a residential home. She didn't turn up for respite care yesterday."

CJ: "How do you feel about that?"
Karen: "Very pleased for Joy and Wilf. The stress is removed from them. Mavis had been getting up three times during the night. They have a different stress now, whether they have made the right decision – '*is* Mum happy there?'. At least they have their home again, plus Joy's own health problems have worsened. It will now be easier for her to cope with this."
CJ: "How would you feel if she wasn't happy there?"
Karen: "I don't know, I may keep in touch with Joy and Wilf."
CJ: "To support them?"
Karen: "Yes."
CJ: "So, accepting some form of ongoing responsibility?"
Karen: "That's the issue – when do you stop?"
CJ: "Yes, clarifying your professional responsibility. You need to unwrap yourself from this involvement. Now the work for you is to close relationships – how to deal with that. Part of closing any relationship is having the opportunity to talk through issues. I believe this is important for you because you have become so involved with Joy and this has left you with a

cocktail of conflicting emotions. Can you be gracious and accept their need to love you?"
Karen: "Yes. I can accept that now."

Commentary

Establishing her personal boundaries in therapeutic relationships was new work for Karen. Yet, looking back, she felt an immense sense of achievement despite her struggle to remain tuned in to both Joy and Mavis. She had realised the hospital philosophy of what it meant to know a person and respond appropriately and she dealt with the emotions and ethical tensions this created. As Menzies-Lyth (1988) stated:

> 'The core of the anxiety situation for the nurse lies in her relation with the patient. The closer and more concentrated this relationship, the more the nurse is likely to experience this anxiety.' (p. 51)

Karen could relate to these words. Ironically and yet profoundly, as practitioners allow themselves to become more involved with patients and became more skilled at managing self within such relationships, caring becomes more valued and satisfying. Without doubt, becoming involved with Mavis and Joy caused anxiety for Karen. Guided reflection helped her to make sense of the unfolding situation and to know herself in ways that enabled her to manage her involvement at an appropriate level. Menzies-Lyth (1988) noted that:

> 'A necessary psychological task for the entrant into any profession that works with people is the development of adequate professional detachment.' (p. 54)

I would restate this as 'adequate professional involvement'. Carmack (1997) asserted that:

> 'Caregivers must learn to balance their engagement with detachment ... to enable caregivers to be present for others while still meeting their own needs ... essential for providing ongoing compassionate effective care.' (p. 139)

Carmack worked with 14 professional and lay caregivers to understand this concept of balance. Using a grounded theory approach, Carmack identified that balancing engagement with detachment was influenced by four factors:

(1)   maintaining consciousness and pragmatism;
(2)   setting limits and boundaries;
(3)   self-monitoring;
(4)   self care.

Maintaining consciousness and pragmatism, setting limits and boundaries are all managed within the existential dialogue. Maintaining consciousness, self-monitoring and self-care require the balance with self made conscious and pragmatic through Karen's dialogue. She identified that a key factor in maintaining the balance was for practitioners to relinquish responsibility for the outcome. Carmack noted:

'Participants said they had had to learn that although they could make a difference to caregiving they could not *fix* people or situations.' (p. 141)

Karen was anxious to fix it for Joy and Wilf, although less so for Mavis. As such Karen needed to learn to let go of responsibility for Joy and Mavis's future. The key was in the dialogue between them, enabling Mavis and Joy to make decisions for themselves. Her role was to help the family make informed decisions. Carmack identified that almost all her respondents had been overinvolved at some point and had suffered the consequences and learning to cope was a 'continually changing process over time'.

Using transactional analysis to pattern self with other

A reason why Karen resisted Joy and Wilf's love was because she felt smothered. Hence, I described her as a rebellious child, resisting her parent's love. A reflective way to help the practitioner see the pattern of communication between herself and other people is through transactional analysis (TA). TA offers the practitioner a framework for viewing patterns of communication between self and others, based on the theory that people communicate from different ego state levels of child (C), adult (A) or parent (P). The child ego state can include a conforming or rebellious child. The adult is associated with the growth of responsibility and reason. The parent is associated with authority; this may be the nurturing or critical parent. When people become anxious they tend to go into script; in other words, they revert to habitual ego state level in order to manage their anxiety (Stewart & Joines, 1987).

Effective communication, although not necessarily therapeutic communication, takes place from reciprocated ego state levels: for example, parent–child, adult–adult. When the pattern of communication is not reciprocated then lines literally become crossed and communication breaks down (Box 6.2). The intention is always to communicate at the most appropriate therapeutic level. From a *working with* perspective, this would usually be adult–adult, although the patient or family may respond from either the child or parent script as a consequence of anxiety or need for comfort and control.

To respond appropriately, the practitioner must read this pattern in the other and manage her own anxiety to prevent herself from slipping into script and responding in either parent or child ego state.

Box 6.2 Reciprocal and non-reciprocal patterns within TA.

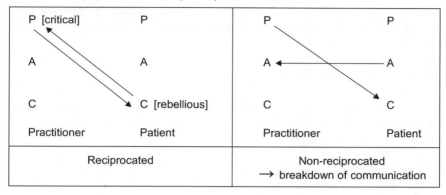

| Reciprocated | Non-reciprocated → breakdown of communication |

In guided reflection I help the practitioner to reflect on both the actual and desirable TA pattern of communication between herself and her patients using the TA analysis reflective framework (Box 6.3). A number of cues are offered to guide the practitioner's reflection.

Box 6.3 Transactional analysis reflective framework.

Plot the pattern of parent/adult/child communication being presented

Actual		**Desirable**	
P Nurturing Critical	P Nurturing Critical	P Nurturing Critical	P Nurturing Critical
A	A	A	A
C Rebellious Conforming	C Rebellious Conforming	C Rebellious Conforming	C Rebellious Conforming
Self	Other	Self	Other

Cues:
- Is the actual pattern therapeutic?
- What factors drew both self and other into this pattern of communication?
- Has this been a repetitive pattern?
- What pattern is desirable (plot on the right side of the chart)?
- What do you need to do to move to this new pattern?

Use the TA analysis reflective framework to reflect on some of your patients and your own patterns of communication with patients. If the pattern is undesirable, see if you can shift the pattern to become more therapeutic.

REFLECTIVE EXEMPLAR 6.5: SID

Sid was 90 and suffered from advanced dementia. He was admitted for frequent respite care. He became extremely anxious and agitated when separated from his daughter.

Karen: "Sid is getting a lot frailer and more childlike now."
CJ: "Less mobile?"
Karen: "He's very unsteady on his feet."
CJ: "What do his carers feel about him?"
Karen: "They've established a routine – for example, to manage his incontinence recently and his agitation. They want us to follow that. His daughter says he's frailer and his chest is still bad."
CJ: "Is it easy to maintain the routines – that everybody follows?"
Karen: "I've put his daughter's letter that explains it all in the notes for everybody to follow."
CJ: "Is he distressed?"
Karen: "No, not as much as usual. He's much weaker."
CJ: "Just burning out?"
Karen: "Yes... It's difficult at times not to mother him now."
CJ: "Do you think that you shouldn't mother him?"
Karen: "To a certain extent. It would be easy to take over from him and not to let him do the things that he can still do."
CJ: "Do you feel sad for him?"
Karen: "Yes."
CJ: "Does he know you?"
Karen: "Yes [laughs]. He says, 'Do I know you?', pointing his fingers at you. I feel sad for him when he comes to tell you that he's going to the toilet and then he has an accident before he gets to use it. We have positioned his bed near the toilet so he can get there easily but he still comes to tell us first."
CJ: "Do you think he's disturbed by his incontinence?"
Karen: "The other day, he didn't even know he had been incontinent."
CJ: "Do you think that was because he didn't want you to know or that he was embarrassed?"
Karen: "I didn't get that impression. I got the impression he had finished and wanted to pull his trousers up."
CJ: "This is an example of how you can look at a situation in different ways. A difficulty with a person with dementia is really knowing what he feels and thinks."

Karen: "My Nan had dementia and I can see what happened to Nan happening to Sid."

CJ: "Does that make it easier or harder, or no difference in caring for Sid?"

Karen: "I don't know, it just hit me. Maybe that's why I feel maternal towards him?"

'Mothering'

I have used the being available template (see Box 4.1) to understand the pattern of relationship between Karen and Sid.

Knowing what is desirable and concern

Karen is concerned with Sid, yet in what I might construe a maternal sense. She illustrates both emotional and control impasses (Ramos, 1992). Hence her concern might be criticised for being misplaced, i.e. not focused on Sid's real needs. Yet what are his real needs? Is Karen aware of the ideology of holistic practice in context of working with patients experiencing dementia and their families?

Knowing Sid

Sid has dementia which makes reading his pattern difficult. Karen sought to interpret the signs, informed by his daughter and her experience of knowing him. From a respite care perspective, it is important to know Sid in context of his normal life pattern in order not to disrupt these patterns. Does she know Sid well enough?

Responding with appropriate action

Karen's 'maternal' stance was a response to Sid's dependence and his 'boy-like' behaviour. Clearly Sid could not respond as a rational adult. Karen needs to tune into Sid's balance of real and potential autonomy, which becomes the focus for knowing who Sid is. However, Karen must also balance Sid's needs with the needs of his family, as he has to go home again. There is evidence that respite care can be very disruptive for the carer's normal management of Sid at home (Dawson, 1987).

Concern and knowing self

Karen's concern for Sid was tinged with sadness and pity for Sid's helplessness. The balance between pity and compassion is fine, as is the balance between instinctual and deliberate parent–child patterns of communication. Yet pity was not helpful because it was based on Karen's own discomfort, as evidenced by the comparison she drew with her grand mother. Karen needed help to work through these feelings towards a feeling of compassion, based on empathy, where she could imagine what it was like for Sid in order to understand and respond to his needs and connect with him through love and understanding. This is not to deny Karen's feelings of pity but to help her understand why she felt this way and to help her grow through these feelings to become the compassionate healer. Without this vision, mothering can easily become smothering, leading to personal distress and blurring of therapeutic intent.

Karen suggested that being protective was a form of emotional entanglement, where she became anxious that others were not responding to Sid 'properly'. The risk was that she could project this absorbed distress as anger at other staff when they were insensitive.

REFLECTIVE EXEMPLAR 6.6: TROY AND LIAM

Karen compared her relationship with Sid to two other male patients, Troy and Liam, whom she felt she had 'mothered'. Troy was recovering from a severe depression, having been transferred from the local psychiatric hospital, whilst Liam was recovering from a severe stroke. Their common denominator was enforced dependence on support to manage everyday activities.

Karen's intuitive response was that mothering was wrong.

Karen: "I know I still do it."
CJ: "Can you make sense of that?"
Karen: "Not really."
CJ: "Do you think the way you care makes you feel that way?"
Karen: "Yes, it could be. But why don't I feel that way with more of the patients?"
CJ: "Is it with a certain type of patient?"
Karen: "I can't see the link between Sid, Troy and Liam. Troy and Liam were both here for rehabilitation – I wanted them to do well, but with Sid, I suppose I still want him to do well."
CJ: "They are not patients you feel particularly close to?"
Karen: "No, not really."
CJ: "Or are they patients who are particularly dependent on you? For example, Troy acted like a little boy unable to do things. Sid responds well to affection. Liam?"
Karen: "I think Liam was the only patient I was getting satisfaction from and maybe that's where the affection comes from."
CJ: "You had a close relationship with Liam's wife?"
Karen: "Yes, she used to come and find me."
CJ: "Do you see mothering as a strength or weakness?"

Karen: "I don't know. Some ways a strength, a reflection of involvement. In other ways, if I give so much to some patients will others suffer?"
CJ: "Perhaps we can link it to a sense of responsibility. For example, Liam is unable to speak, dress, feed himself, is incontinent, frightened and determined, yet responsive and vulnerable – like a child growing up. Troy is like a child unable to dress himself, find the toilet, yet always charming and grateful – like a good little boy. Sid is hopelessly confused but always full of fun and laughing – very dependent on you, like a little boy. And all are men."

We explored Karen's sense of responsibility to each of these three patients. The outcome was that the greater the responsibility, the greater the involvement. Karen framed her relationships with each of these men within PAC ego states and how she had perceived each as a child so the instinct was to respond as the parent.

Karen linked this insight to her anger when Elizabeth (a patient) had insisted on calling her 'Karie'. Karen had perceived this as being treated like a child. Karen reflected that her response had been like an angry adolescent wanting to be acknowledged as a grown-up. This resulted in avoidance, which led to a breakdown in her relationship with Elizabeth.

Mothering was Karen's deep subconscious reaction to the men's dependence. I challenged Karen to reflect on whether these ego state communications were therapeutic. My challenge was based on the concept of symbiosis – how communication can become stuck within a self-perpetuating pattern of ego state communication in which two or more people behave as though they are one person. In Karen's relationships with these three men, this symbiosis was demonstrated by her moving between her parent and adult ego states whilst encouraging the men to stay within their child ego state. This symbiosis was both comfortable and satisfying for Karen and she had also assumed, albeit subconsciously, that it was comfortable for her patients. As such, each was motivated to maintain this communication state. Maintaining the parent ego state was a coping strategy by which Karen could control her environment. However, except for Sid, its therapeutic value could be challenged. As part of their rehabilitation, Liam and Troy needed to be helped to accept responsibility.

Perhaps this helped to explain why Karen got so angry when patients reduced her to the child role. It illustrated how self's concerns can decrease the ability to interpret the clinical situation in terms of the patient's needs and subsequently reduce the ability of the practitioner to 'be available'.

REFLECTIVE EXEMPLAR 6.7: ELIZABETH

Karen had shared her frustration at working with Elizabeth in an earlier guided reflection session with me. She felt Elizabeth treated her like a child, especially in front of her relatives.

Karen: "I've been through reasons for feeling like that, but I'm left feeling the same way. Reading the Morse paper (1991), I could make sense of it as one of the steps of building up relationships. I've not experienced that before – it really affected me at the time."

CJ: "And that feeling has passed now?"

Karen: "Yes, but I don't feel I coped with it particularly well. I've never got that close to a patient before . . . I tried to make sense of why she was doing it, but I didn't get anywhere. I gave her feedback that I didn't like the nicknames, that they embarrassed me – things like 'angel of delight', 'Karie'."

CJ: "And did she stop?"

Karen: "She said she would but she didn't."

CJ: "Do you think she was trying to mother you?"

Karen: "To some extent. I don't need mothering – I'm qualified now. They still see me as a 22-year-old girl!"

CJ: "Can you see that she may have had a need to mother you as her way of coping?"

Karen: "If she was like that then wouldn't she act that way with some of the other staff?"

CJ: "She may not want to mother everyone. She may just want to mother you."

Karen: "I felt I didn't want to go near her if she was going to be like this."

CJ: "Did you feel like giving her that feedback?"

Karen acknowledged her embarrassment and discomfort at this: "I wondered whether she was feeling superior to the other patients or whether she was totally innocent, and that she wasn't aware of what she was doing."

CJ: "Or that was her way of coping?"

Karen: "Yes. Her family are all like that as well."

CJ: "She's being transferred back here in two days. You need to explore it with her and work out this tension. Otherwise you will be unavailable to her and not able to use yourself therapeutically to work with her."

Karen: "That's exactly what I've written!"

CJ: "So, what have we said – what are the issues?"

Karen: "Elizabeth doesn't seem to want criticism – doesn't want challenging – wants support for herself as she is now."

CJ: "And you are reluctant to give Elizabeth support on her terms and reluctant to confront her because you want to protect her and yourself?"

Karen: "I really should have stopped it first time it happened but I didn't know how it was going to affect me."

CJ: "Perhaps the skill is to know yourself so you frame these issues in terms of understanding the other's need, in contrast with taking it personally. We have seen on previous occasions how this blurs the therapeutic intent Having this conversation, do you think you'll act differently towards her?"

Karen: "Yes."

Knowing self

A moment of deep insight for Karen – that to be available to the patient, she needed to understand the underlying reasons why the patient responded as she did and to understand her own reaction to this behaviour. Karen's confrontation had been ineffective. She had wanted to be the critical parent, to tell Elizabeth off for her 'naughty' behaviour. When this failed she responded as a 'hurt' child, withdrawn and sulky.

People cope with anxiety in hospital in different ways. It was important for Karen to see the underlying reasons for Elizabeth's actions or feel confident enough to confront her with her unacceptable behaviour. Karen indicated her caution in using confrontation skills because she associated these with being uncaring and with potential conflict. Yet this was because confrontation was motivated by her emotional reaction rather than as a therapeutic response to Elizabeth.

Use the TA framework to reflect on your own patterns of communication with patients, relatives and colleagues. Are these patterns therapeutic?

Knowing and managing self is fundamental to being available to work with the patient and family to help them meet their health needs. Yet we also need to create caring environments that facilitate being available. Creating and sustaining an adequate caring environment is the essence of Chapter 7.

Chapter 7

Creating an Environment to Support Holistic Practice

Introduction

The practitioner's ability to be available to work with the patient and family is influenced to a great extent by the conditions of practice. The nurse–patient relationship is always contextualised in terms of a real world that may constrain the practitioner's ability to give effective and desirable care; factors embodied within self or perceived as embedded within the health-care environment. Embodied factors might include such issues as being unassertive, being burnt out, being fearful of speaking out, stress and difficult relationships with other nurses and doctors. Embedded factors might include such resource issues as the establishment and skill mix, workload, support systems, management style and leadership.

A general perception is that caring is not valued within organisations, beyond rhetoric. It behoves the practitioner to take appropriate action towards creating conditions where being available is possible. Yet caring may be difficult to assert within a culture of managerialism that has focused organisations to become lean and driven to meet medically determined outcomes for minimum cost. As such, nursing is often regarded as a soft asset to strip because:

- its processes and outcomes are marginal to purchasing plans;
- it has an extensive workforce and represents a significant slice of the budget;
- it does not have a strong voice within the organisational culture;
- it regulates itself as a subordinate and powerless group controlled by an internalised threat of sanction.

As Ray (1989) noted:

'The transformation of health care systems to corporate enterprises emphasising competitive management and economic gains seriously challenges nursing's humanistic philosophies and theories and nursing's administrative and clinical practices.' (p. 31)

Shifting norms

Conditions of practice can be internalised – 'This is the way we do things round here'. The power of these conditions constitutes norms or normal ways of going about things. Norms are the taken-for-granted structures that determine ways of relating to people which are embedded and reinforced in everyday actions. Because they are normal, they are rarely reflected on for their significance in achieving desirable work. Consider when you last commenced a new post or reflect on how new staff are very conscious of fitting in and being accepted as normal. People who don't fit in are quickly targeted as misfits and pressure is brought to bear on them to toe the party line.

Hence conditions of practice or norms are powerful and not easy to shift, especially as they constitute what is usually described as the *status quo*. Yet a shift of norms is essential to create and sustain an environment to support caring in practice. Practitioners need to consider the conditions of practice that might prevent them realising the philosophy within everyday practice (see Box 1.2). Within this process practitioners must inevitably become 'politically oriented', accepting a commitment to take action to create the conditions in which caring can be realised. Consider again the reflective process of enlightenment, empowerment, and emancipation (Box 3.1):

- understanding the conditions of practice and the way these limit achieving desirable work;
- being empowered to take action to change these conditions;
- changing conditions resulting in the achievement of desirable work.

Understanding the conditions of practice is like peeling back layers to reveal the norms that determine culture.

Box 7.1 sets out the shift of norms I feel are necessary to support holistic practice (Johns, 1998a). This offers a reflective framework to challenge and guide the practitioner to consider the impact of these norms within her own practice and to consider how these norms can be shifted in order to realise desirable and effective practice.

Perhaps you have been challenged by the earlier chapters to reflect on your own belief system and whether your beliefs are adequately represented in your philosophy for practice and whether they are contradicted within practice. Perhaps you have also reflected on the way you manage work and whether it is congruent with working with patients and families from a holistic perspective. Consider the extent to which your own practice fits with the norms concerned with coping and support. Do you accept responsibility to establish an environment of mutual support in which you and your colleagues are available to each other in ways that parallel being available to patients and families? Are you sensitive to the stress of your colleagues? Do

Box 7.1   The movement from old norms to new, congruent with holistic practice.

Movement from old norms	$\longrightarrow$	Towards new norms
Belief system Nursing-centred belief system – medical perspective of knowing what's best for the patient	$\longrightarrow$	Patient-centred belief system – concerned with holistic practice working with patients
Managing work Managing delegated work based on task-centred practice and getting through the work within shifts	$\longrightarrow$	Managing work based on individual responsibility and knowing and responding to individual needs

Coping and support
Good nurses cope by:
• maintaining a facade of
  competence
• use of incongruent ways of
  defending self
	$\longrightarrow$	Accepting responsibility to
		establish an environment of
		mutual support in which
		staff are available to each
		other

Power Perceiving self as powerless, dependent and responding in hierarchical ways	$\longrightarrow$	Accepting role responsibility to ensure desirable work as a process of collaboration with others

you support your colleagues well enough? Do you get adequate support at work? How might this be improved? What factors limit practitioners being available to support each other at work? Can these factors be overcome?

In the reflective exemplar below, George's story, Karen is an associate nurse practitioner at Burford. She strongly believe in holistic practice as set out in Box 1.2. Note the emphasis on collaborative ways of working written in the Burford philosophy. Practitioners at Burford chose to organise the delivery of care through primary nursing because it would seem to facilitate the nurse–patient relationship. Primary nursing would also facilitate collaborative ways of relating between practitioners working together towards meeting patient need. Collaboration is espoused as desirable but what does collaboration mean in practice? It must mean a de-emphasis on bureaucratic hierarchical ways of relating by focusing on individual and collective responsibility between practitioners that cuts across professional interests and traditional ways of relating. As you read through this chapter, reflect on the extent to which norms congruent with holistic practice have been realised in the reflective exemplars and within your own practice.

REFLECTIVE EXEMPLAR 7.1: GEORGE'S STORY

In George's story, Karen illustrates the significance of confronting her own and others' responsibility to see and respond to George as a person. George is a regular respite care patient who was perceived by all staff, including Karen, as a 'difficult patient' because of his crudity and attention-seeking behaviour. As a consequence, staff were motivated to avoid George, rationalising their non-availability to him in terms of his socially unacceptable behaviour.

> *Karen*: "George – I've done some work with him. I made an effort during his last admission to spend time with him to make him feel he doesn't bore people. As a consequence, my whole opinion of him changed. I found him to be lonely, frightened of dying and actually found him to be quite receptive to some suggestions and opinions. I was really glad that I did that because other people's opinions of George had influenced me from the start."
> *CJ*: "Negatively, I take it."
> *Karen*: "Yes. In the notes I challenged everyone's behaviour towards George, although nobody has read it yet. I wrote it on Sunday and he was discharged on Monday morning."
> *CJ*: "What is the significance?"
> *Karen*: "How strongly other people's opinions influence you."
> *CJ*: "Have you kept a distance from him before?"
> *Karen*: "Yes. I always made an excuse to get away."
> *CJ*: "Which is what others do?"
> *Karen*: "They stand at the foot of the bed – they don't sit down next to him."
> *CJ*: "Which is what you did as well?"
> *Karen*: "I challenged myself as well in the notes."

I noted the value of role modelling to encourage people to look at themselves. They are more likely to look at themselves when they see that Karen had also challenged herself.

> *CJ*: "It's so important to see through our own limited perceptions of people if we are going to help them."
> *Karen*: "It reinforced the value of time, like with Mrs Kitchen. I wouldn't have discussed her fear with her or spent time with George if I hadn't had time to sit and listen to him."
> *CJ*: "It's not just time but how we choose to use it, to choose to use it in that way. Time you would have spent doing something else. This is a good example of realising the significance of 'situated meaning' as reflected in the unit's philosophy – to understand where George is coming from. It sounds a very powerful experience."
> *Karen*: "I felt very tall. It made me see how therapeutic it was for all people

involved – including me. I was working with Carolyn [care assistant] that evening. She often has an unacceptable attitude towards patients. I showed her what I had written about George. She read what I had written and made an effort with him that evening."

CJ: "Did that warm her to you?"

Karen: "I've warmed to her a lot, just as I have with George, and give her more credit than others do."

CJ: "Are your impressions of Carolyn based on what others have told you?"

Karen: 'I found that out for myself that she was not easy to work with. She had a brusque manner with patients, but by going deeper I found a different Carolyn."

CJ: "So that was a real bonus for you. Do you enjoy working with her now?"

Karen: "Yes, whereas before I dreaded working with her, especially after an episode when she had upset Rita [a patient] and made her feel like a little child. I told Carolyn that she should have apologised and she said, 'No way I would apologise'. It's given me the strength to challenge people's opinions. I would defend Carolyn now, to get people to think about the positive sides of people."

In a later session Karen said: "I noticed that Gayle [primary nurse] had the 'old attitude'. I should have pointed out the notes to her. It says things like 'he's lonely' and 'he's frightened'. I felt miffed that the notes were not picked up on, but I didn't want to thrust it under people's noses. I wanted them to come back to me on it."

CJ: "How could you be more effective?"

Karen: "I could sit down with the staff and say, 'Don't you think you could...'"

Drawing on Heron's six-category intervention analysis (Box 5.2), I responded: "What do you think about using a cathartic intervention? For example, you could say to particular staff at handover, 'How do you find George?' or 'Does George wind you up?'. This may create the opportunity for other staff to express their feelings about George. This would confront their own reaction to George and lead into reorientating care in terms of George's needs and discussing what you've written."

Karen: "I can accept how others feel, but it did take a lot of energy to find the new George."

CJ: "What are you saying?"

Karen: "I suppose I'm saying I'm letting their attitude ride because I understand how they feel and why I didn't challenge them. I can see he has upset people in the past therefore people genuinely have a block to forming a good relationship with him. You can't be therapeutic with everyone."

CJ: "Is that position okay?"

Karen: "It was this time, but I did think that during his next admission that as no-one commented on what I had found out six weeks or three months ago, I will ask if they had read my notes and thought about it this admission. A couple of the care assistants read the notes."
CJ: "Did you get feedback from them?"
Karen: "No. I must do that. I'll ask them this evening. Thinking about it, Tricia did seem much more willing to understand him afterwards."

Commentary

Karen illustrated that the space needed to see George involved clearing away her own preconceptions and prejudices, which had resulted in labelling George as difficult, with the consequence that she had not been available to work with him. This experience was a transformative moment for Karen. For the first time she really knew the meaning of the unit's philosophy and her therapeutic potential.

Karen drew a parallel between George and Carolyn, who was also known in terms of her 'difficult' behaviour. Karen dreaded working with Carolyn; it was energy draining for Karen. Infused with new energy from her affirming experience with George, Karen responded positively to Carolyn.

Consider why Carolyn was so responsive to Karen's feedback. Do you work with colleagues whose attitudes are non-caring? If you avoid confronting this attitude or behaviour, how does that make you feel? What do you need to do and how can you do it?

Karen challenged Carolyn's behaviour in ways that did not result in Carolyn's defensive aggression. The key was to shift her energy from negative to positive. This enabled her to break a repetitive cycle of anxiety in working with a difficult colleague and patient. Karen also felt elated, illustrating the satisfaction and joy of caring and its impact on neutralising anxiety. The secret of confrontation was by role modelling rather than direct confrontation. Responding to George in positive ways allowed him to reduce his need to act out to seek attention. He was now known. Consequently, George was not so negatively labelled and less anxious.

Karen had acted out her role responsibility to create collaborative ways of working; this resulted in Karen and Carolyn being more available to support each other. Yet Karen felt reluctant to confront more senior colleagues. As such, she sacrificed her responsibility both to George to ensure he received congruent care, and to her colleagues to work towards collaborative relationships. She saw that her failure to assert George's needs adversely affected the care he received. Karen's concern about upsetting her colleagues was always bubbling on the surface of this experience. She tried to cope with this contradiction between supporting the staff and advocating for George by rationalising the staff's reaction to him. She did not want to thrash a lost cause or unnecessarily create conflict with her colleagues. However, she anticipated the future positively in her resolve to confront her colleagues when George was next admitted.

Some seven months later, Karen shared a further experience concerning George.

Karen: "George is in now. He has been here since the beginning of December. He's had a 'Jacksonian' fit. It primarily affects one side. His hand is totally useless. A nursing home is being found for him. Whereas I used to feel good about him, I realise a main reason for that was that he was going home after a week's respite care. Now that he's here for that much longer, I get very tired, and lose my rag at him like everybody else does. I feel sad about that."

CJ: "You say 'I get very tired' – do you mean generally or with him?"

Karen: "Tired of him – he thinks he's at death's door and wants our attention even more. I'm tired of his buzzer sounding."

CJ: "Because you have developed a positive relationship with him, can you give him feedback?"

Karen: "Yes!! And that's the good thing. I *can* be honest with him."

CJ: "But that's not enough?"

Karen: "I find things . . . like he's got a Doctor Jekyll and Hyde personality. They seem to have a real problem with him on nights and whereas in the past, in the mornings, they could tell me, I would say, 'Is it this, is it that', now I don't . . . I've had enough of hearing about it."

CJ: "Are you denying the night staff the opportunity to offload?"

Karen: "Not that. I *do* listen but I don't have the energy to do anything about it."

CJ: "Perhaps the night staff make him like that?"

Karen: "Gayle and I thought that might be so. Then Fay [associate nurse] worked a night. She confirmed he was absolutely different at night."

I acknowledged Karen's feelings: "I think you should still be involved with George. You don't want to throw that away?"

Karen: "No, not at all."

Commentary

Karen was in a stressful dilemma, being battered by the demands of caring yet unable to reject George to save herself because of her concern for him. It highlighted the boundaries of personal tolerance. That she sometimes struggled to manage her own concerns was a reflection of her humanness. Her concern has been nurtured yet now her concern felt battered, at risk, leaving her in a constant dilemma between her concern to care and coping with the effort. She needed support from her colleagues rather than to feel frustrated at them because of their persistent uncaring attitude towards George.

Some four months later Karen talked through her feelings about George's death.

> *Karen*: "George – he died when I was on annual leave. I was amazed at myself when I heard the news. I felt real grief for him. In the past I had felt very sad for patients, but with George, I identified similar feelings for him as I would for a member of my family. It made me think of things – 'I wish I hadn't said that, wish I had done this'. It brought home how much that relationship had meant to me. I had seen it as learning but had not seen quite how much it mattered to me."
>
> *CJ*: "I knew it would be tough for you. Do you know the circumstances of his death?"
>
> *Karen*: "He died because he gave up. He saw no future. He said it wasn't very positive, yet he still had control over his life to the very end."
>
> *CJ*: "Can you put your feelings for George into perspective?"
>
> *Karen*: "Grief. I was very attached to him, there was a closeness between us."
>
> *CJ*: "And how are you dealing with it."
>
> *Karen*: "Still very sad. But identifying these feelings has helped the process to complete itself."
>
> *CJ*: "The consequences of human encounter and therapeutic work. And yet they are also the sources of satisfaction."
>
> *Karen*: "I see that. I don't know how I would cope with a greater number of patients if I was a primary nurse."
>
> *CJ*: "It highlights your need to be skilled at managing your feelings whilst remaining available to George. If you were George's primary nurse you would have probably felt more in control of the relationship. Perhaps some of your grief is not having been able to take the best action for George; for example, when you last talked about his care, you were very frustrated at your own actions and the actions of others. There are many factors that led you to become close to George – labelling and rejection of him by others; his complexity and vulnerability, and struggle for respect; cutting your therapeutic teeth on him; his sudden death, you being on holiday, not being able to say good-bye well enough."

The therapeutic team

Sharing this experience was a profound moment of realisation for Karen as she acknowledged her sadness as a reflection of the human encounter that comes with concern and involvement. Talking through her feelings helped Karen to honour George, to work through any guilt and to recognise the joy that caring for George brought her. The moment was transformative for Karen. Yet it was critical that she was guided in this moment. For relatively inexperienced, yet sensitive and caring nurses such as Karen, it is important to acknowledge and work though personal feelings of grief. A patient's death can be traumatic for the practitioner. Sustaining caring in practice requires practitioners to mutually care for each other in ways that parallel their caring endeavour with patients and families. It sounds so simple – that nurses should be available to each other for mutual support. And yet in practice it seems so hard to realise. Why is this? Is it because when practitioners are anxious, they retreat into flight and fight modes necessary for survival? If so, then it may require another person, empathic and sensitive to the other's situation, to respond, 'I can see this is tough for you'. Try this out with a colleague. The impact can be remarkable.

Perhaps, as practitioners, we are not good at being available for each other. Practitioners may avoid 'being available' opportunities with their colleagues because of the 'good nurses cope' syndrome Nurses may rationalise their failure to seek help as not wanting to burden their colleagues. Jade noted that she felt guilty about seeking support from her colleagues because it put pressure on them: 'I've tried to use other people more rather than saving things up but I don't want to burden other people' (Johns, 1998a, p. 206).

Street (1992) describes this phenomenon as 'partial visibility', whereby nurses cope with their practice by being partially invisible to each other. Street (1992) believes that this is related to the inability of staff to give negative feedback in a constructive manner and leads to a non-recognition of distress in nurses by other nurses. Karen was frustrated by her colleagues who failed to follow planned care or give her feedback. She was saying 'I am visible' as others tried to mask their visibility. Practitioners who aim to be invisible do not go about seeking feedback to monitor their own effectiveness. They are also defensive to feedback from others, fearing criticism. As a consequence, they also become unable to support each other, wrapped up in their own defensive self-concern.

Given the significance of staff caring for each other to support the caring quest, practitioners need to find ways to break down the barriers that sustain a culture of 'invisibility' in order to become available to each other for mutual support. This is the essence of the therapeutic team. Support for the therapeutic team is offered by Vachon (1987):

'The most effective antidote for the alleviation and prevention of stress . . . had to do with a sense of team philosophy, team support and team building.' (p. 157)

Norbeck (1985) found that social support from fellow nurses was the most effective way to reduce stress. Yet, as the stories have suggested, this type of team is not easy to develop, suggesting that practitioners' ability to care for each other has not been nurtured within practice environments. The stories illustrate the way reflection can expose these norms and promote action to shift the norms to support a culture of mutual caring. Within a reflective culture based on responsibility, caring and strong leadership, reflective opportunities can constantly challenge and undermine inappropriate norms whilst reinforcing caring relationships between colleagues based on mutual responsibility.

Consider your own practice. Do you avoid sharing your feelings? Do you avoid dealing with conflict? Has reflection enabled you to become more visible, more authentic and caring with your colleagues?

Debriefing

Mutual support can be facilitated by encouraging practitioners to share their experiences with their colleagues and to debrief particular incidents that cause anxiety and distress. Such opportunity exists on a daily basis in hospitals, at ward meetings and handover situations. This may be more difficult to facilitate in community settings where clinical leadership is uncertain but regular meetings can be arranged for this purpose.

It is likely that if one practitioner is angry or distressed about a situation, then others will be as well. Debriefing can also be about celebrating satisfaction and joy, acknowledging and valuing success and caring. The benefits of debriefing are summarised in Box 7.2.

Box 7.2   The benefits of debriefing.

Reflective debriefing creates an opportunity:

- For individual practitioners to get support; to give practitioners a 'voice' to be heard above the din, to be recognised and valued as people with human needs and human frailties.
- For staff to share feelings. Debriefing sets up a norm that it is okay to be angry or distressed and to share these feelings and cuts across a culture where practitioners have hidden their feelings in the belief that 'good nurses cope' and do not burden their colleagues.
- To bring staff together for mutual support and constructing the 'desirable' therapeutic team.
- To confront inappropriate attitudes/behaviour/defence mechanisms that prevent practitioners realising holistic practice.
- For clinical leaders to role model the disclosure of feelings and to encourage and facilitate reflection in others.
- To create a 'space' in a busy world that acknowledges the significance of support in practice and prioritises this aspect of practice.
- To make visible and reinforce caring values.
- To promote the morale, motivation and self-esteem of staff, with the organisational consequences of retaining staff, enhancing quality of practice and reducing staff sickness.
- To learn through experience to manage self better in subsequent situations.

Accepting role responsibility to ensure adequate support

A potential problem with guided reflection or clinical supervision is that stressful situations are saved up to share in the session, which may discourage practitioners from dealing with anxiety and energy-draining feelings within everyday practice. Imagine that your next supervision session is three weeks away. Do you live with the stress until then or take action to seek appropriate support now? Try saying at hand over, 'I am struggling with my feelings about. . .'. Accept responsibility for getting your own support.

As a reflective practitioner, I accept responsibility for ensuring that patients and families receive the most appropriate care. As such, I need to be in the best possible shape to be available to my patients and families. As Karen illustrated in her work with George, this may mean confronting inappropriate attitudes and care by colleagues. It also means challenging the wider organisation on its policies that impact negatively on patient care. However, as Karen illuminated, the difficulty of confrontation should not be under estimated because she feared the negative reaction of those she perceived as more powerful others.

Sources of power

Hierarchy is a powerful intimidator because it works on positional, sanction and reward power (Box 7. 3). French & Raven's categories of power offer the practitioner a useful reflective technique to consider their own and others' use of power within any situation. Consider a situation when you have wanted to confront a more senior nurse but didn't. Why was that? Collaborative relationships are based on relational and expert power; that is why Carolyn (p. 166) changed her attitude and behaviour. Yet Karen needed to feel powerful enough to take that action. She felt disempowered to challenge more senior colleagues.

Managing conflict

Many practitioners like Karen are reticent about sharing experiences of conflict in a culture where talking about colleagues is akin to 'telling tales'. The root of all conflict is found in differences of beliefs, values and power. Remind yourself of the way ethical mapping guides the practitioner to reflect on conflict, values and authority to resolve dilemmas (see Box 5.1). Interpersonal conflict is the most common focus for shared experience within guided reflection (Johns, 1996b). Vachon (1987) drew similar conclusions from her sample of 581 caregivers from a variety of countries, health-care professions and settings. She noted:

Box 7.3 Leadership and sources of power (French & Raven, 1968).

Hierarchical emphasis of power	Collaborative emphasis of power
Reward power Based on the subordinate's perception that the leader has the ability and resources to obtain rewards for those who comply with directives	*Referent power* Based on the subordinate's identification with the leader. The leader exercises influence because of perceived attractiveness, personal characteristics, reputation or what is called 'charisma'
Coercive power Based on fear and the subordinate's perception that the leader has the ability to punish or bring about undesirable outcomes	*Expert power* Based on the subordinate;s perception of the leader as someone who is competent and who has some special knowledge or expertise in a given area
Legitimate power Based on the subordinate's perception that the leader has a right and authority to exercise influence because of the leader's role or position in the organisation.	

'Perhaps unexpectedly, most of the stressors caregivers reported, when asked about the stress they experienced in caring for the critically ill and dying, were not related to work with clients and their families but, rather to difficulties with colleagues and with institutional hierarchies.' (p. 150)

Evidence suggests that nurses primarily use non-assertive methods of managing conflict, either through avoidance or accommodation (Cavanagh, 1991). However, collaboration is a mutual process. It takes two to tango! The practitioner works towards collaborative ways of managing conflict even though the other person may be reluctant to dance! This may often feel like a struggle against the power gradients of more powerful others.

REFLECTIVE EXEMPLAR 7.2: FABRICE

Leslie shared an experience that concerned his ongoing conflict with Rachel, the district nurse.

Leslie: "Rachel came to the hospital for computing work. She looked at the board. I told her that Fabrice was going home next Friday. She identified a range of reasons why he shouldn't go home – such issues as her workload, his wife, is he ready? I explained to her that he was ready to go home. Fabrice appeared at the doorway. He talked to her about his readiness to go home and even she had to admit that he was well prepared. After

Fabrice had gone back to his room she said, 'Thank you very much, that was most enlightening'. I suspect if Fabrice hadn't appeared on cue and hadn't backed up what I said, she wouldn't have been so amenable in her responses to me at the end."

CJ: "Presumably you had discussed the discharge earlier with her?"

Leslie: "Oh yes."

CJ: "Was there a home assessment?"

Leslie: "No, he is self-caring. The complication factor is his invalid wife. I arranged extra support for him with social services. It has all been thought through."

CJ: "So what did Rachel think her input would be?"

Leslie: "She said he would feel inadequately supported at home – in hospital he has 24 hour support, and that he wouldn't manage: 'We don't have the resources in the community'."

CJ: "Do you know what the GP felt?"

Leslie: "Gary said some time ago that Fabrice would know when he was ready to go home – we had all discussed that."

CJ: "That was important knowledge – having that behind you?"

Leslie: "Rachel still has this 'we know best' attitude towards patient care; for example, we know best when it's time for them to go home, taking the responsibility out of their hands, it's reflected in her patronising attitude towards him. I find it difficult to tell her that."

Commentary

Fabrice's own 'voice' was compelling and could not be denied. It refocused the caring moment within Fabrice's needs and highlighted the therapeutic action of involving the patient in negotiating his own care rather than being treated as an object to be cared for. However, Fabrice's intervention was opportunistic; perhaps Leslie should have been more deliberate in involving Fabrice in his discussion/altercation with Rachel, creating the milieu for Fabrice to exercise his autonomy.

Leslie's sense of triumph felt perverse, reflecting his persistent competitive, win–lose relationship with Rachel and the way professional concerns and conflict can obscure what's best for the patient and family.

Horizontal violence

Interpersonal conflict between nurses and possibly between nurses and other professions, but usually excluding doctors, can be viewed as *horizontal violence* (Freire, 1972). Horizontal violence is symptomatic of the way people belonging to oppressed groups might respond to each other in 'violent ways' as a reflection of their alienation from each other and as a consequence of being unable to direct their felt violence toward their powerful oppressors.

Yet often, expression of this violence is muted within the culture of the harmonious team. Within this team, practitioners are motivated to avoid public display of conflict and hostility and project instead an illusion of harmony. The harmonious team is:

'... concerned with maintaining a facade of togetherness or teamwork. It does not talk about difficult feelings between its members and seeks to protect its members from outside threat. Conflict is brushed under the carpet or is inadequately resolved.' (Johns, 1992, pp. 91–92)

Such response is antitherapeutic, as the need to get on with colleagues on a superficial level that avoids direct expression of difficult feelings and conflict is more important than therapeutic work with patients. Clearly, this sort of team cannot support therapeutic work with patients on a holistic level.

REFLECTIVE EXEMPLAR 7.3: HANK'S COMPLAINT

The impact of the harmonious team and horizontal violence is vividly illustrated in an experience Karen shared with me in guided reflection. The risk of giving colleagues feedback that exposes their non-therapeutic responses is that one will be criticised and rejected for not conforming to the norm of the 'harmonious team'. Karen illustrated the consequences of breaking this cultural norm when she 'exposed' a patient's complaint by writing in the patient's notes about the way the care assistant on night duty had treated him.

Karen: "One night last week Hank complained to me about the actions of one of the night staff. He was very angry about it, so I wrote about his complaint in his notes, really to cover my own back because if something had happened because of that – if he had got worked up and had a heart attack. I didn't state who was involved or the nature of the incident. Christine [night associate nurse] picked up what I had written in the notes and said that she felt 'very sad I had to write that – that some things were better said, not written'. She didn't deny the incident but criticised my documenting it."
CJ: "The way you handled it?"
Karen: "Right. I re-read my notes of the incident because I had written them in a hurry. I realised I had used a word that could have been replaced by a better one."
CJ: "An antagonistic word?"
Karen: "Yes. I made a comment further on in the notes and replaced my initial note to make it more clear to people."
CJ: "Less volatile?"
Karen: "Yes, but what got to me was Christine criticising me about my

way of documenting it when the *Nursing Times* goes on about 'whistle blowing' and how complaints should be documented. I felt she was trying to cover for the person involved even though she acknowledged that the event happened."

CJ: "And now?"

Karen: "I pointed it out to Leslie as he was the primary nurse. He commented, 'I'll have a word with the person involved'. I went home and worried about it all night, worried how she would take it, what she would say. So I need feedback."

CJ: "What would you do differently given the same situation again?"

Karen: "Only thing I could have done was to ring her and ask her to explain from her point of view."

CJ: "Think of the response you might have got from this."

Karen: "From my perspective, if it was me – I would have appreciated it."

CJ: "And knowing the person involved?"

Karen: "I can't say. She could nearly be my grandmother."

CJ: "How do you normally get on with her?"

Karen outlined a superficial relationship.

CJ: "Do you think this action was out of character for her?"

Karen: "I think it was an exaggeration of her normal character."

CJ: "You think?"

Karen: "I don't work with her. It's difficult to know how she is with the other patients. The event itself is quite trivial, it's Hank's anger that got to me."

CJ: "Do you think Hank's anger was reasonable?"

Karen: "I felt that at the time I would have been upset and angry. She was inflicting her values on him, not respecting him."

We explored Karen's options. We agreed she should talk this through with the care assistant. This was not possible face to face but she could ring her at home. I asked Karen if she still wanted Leslie to deal with it. She suggested that he didn't want to. Karen felt she hadn't wanted him to do it in the first place, it was because he had offered. We rehearsed Karen's response to the associate nurse, acknowledging that what Karen did was morally correct although an insensitive way for giving feedback. The key factor was to keep the situation grounded in the therapeutic situation rather than becoming a secondary situation of interpersonal conflict. I urged Karen to take action because of her personal integrity even though she was fearful at this prospect.

Commentary

Karen took action to fulfil her responsibility to a patient by confronting the unacceptable actions of a colleague. In doing so, she broke the rule of the harmonious team. As Karen discovered, she became the villain.

Following session

Karen: "I went home and phoned her!"
CJ: "How did you feel when you picked up the telephone receiver?"
Karen: "Terrified – she was angry, but didn't get as angry as she possibly could have done."
CJ: "Have you learnt that it pays to belong to the harmonious team? If so, if a similar situation occurs, you will think twice before confronting it?"
Karen: "Yes."
CJ: "What can you do about it?"
Karen felt dejected.
CJ: "Perhaps share this situation with your other colleagues to secure their support and to assert the therapeutic team to offset this malignancy."
Karen: "I felt like a chicken at the prospect of Leslie acting on my behalf. I'm now feeling humbled. I didn't stop to think. I'm feeling very stupid. Why did Hank wait to see me? He just happened to see me – probably just thinking of it at the time."
CJ: "How do you think Mandy [the care assistant] might be feeling?"
Karen: "I hope she thinks that I had the courage to ring her."
CJ: "Your phone call was a cathartic intervention. You enabled Mandy to vent her anger at you. However, she also knows she did not act appropriately. She did not like being exposed. You can rationalise her anger in this way. You must not see yourself in the wrong."

Despite her distress, Karen said that she enjoyed going through it step by step. She liked least her feelings that she didn't want to come to the session as she thought it was going to be too hard. She had a slight residual fear about further retribution but the care assistant was now on holiday for one month.

Commentary

The issue had degenerated into a secondary issue about Karen breaking social norms by exposing a colleague in this way. Karen had to defend her actions in writing the note, as though it were she who was in the wrong for exposing her colleague in this way. The situation had twisted from being a patient-related issue to being an interpersonal issue. In other words, loyalty to her colleagues took precedence over loyalty to patients.

Karen's distress is a reflection of the power of the harmonious team. Perhaps she was limiting her damage to the harmonious team by accepting her 'villain' role. As she noted, she was learning to play by the rules. Karen was not supported by Hank's primary nurse, who 'forgot' to give Mandy feedback. This reflected the primary nurse's own socialisation within the harmonious team and role failure to act in the patient's best interests. The power of the harmonious team cannot be over-estimated. It is a deeply embedded norm ignored at peril, as Karen learnt. And yet it is the antithesis of the therapeutic team because it is grounded in the best interests of staff rather than patients.

If I had been the line manager and supervisor I would have intervened and confronted Mandy and Christine with their actions and responses. I could have done this legitimately (i.e. not breaking the confidentiality rule of supervision) because it had become a public issue. This is an example of a situation where the practitioner could not take appropriate action on her own and needed more powerful others to help tackle these barriers. By tackling the issues publicly, it might have led to more open ways of managing conflict and inappropriate practice. As it was, the issue was brushed under the carpet as best forgotten, although it would fester into increased break-down of relationships between Karen and the night staff.

On a deeper psychoanalytic level, the harmonious team is a social defence system to protect staff from anxiety. The team maintains an illusion of being caring to each other even though in reality it stifles the expression of feelings and the positive resolution of conflict.

Consider to what extent the existence of this type of team stifles the sharing of feelings and expression and resolution of conflict.

REFLECTIVE EXEMPLAR 7.4: HELEN'S STORY

Consider Helen's experiences with two patients during which she confronted what she perceived to be inappropriate action by other staff, yet in ways that facilitated the development of the therapeutic team. Note also the way she established the existential dialogue with her patients and how this created a conflict of values with her colleagues, leading to a sense of outrage.

Helen: "Am I just a technician? This experience concerned a lady I saw this week. She's about 80, lovely lady, very ill. She was admitted to one of the elderly care wards in early December. She had ruptured her oesophagus – this carries an 80% risk of mortality. Later she had a femoral embolus that required a right above-knee amputation. She was referred to me for total parenteral nutrition [TPN]. The aim was for the oesophagus to heal spontaneously – it can happen. But not with this lady! She had a massive leak into her mediastinum. The doctors with hindsight had some regrets about the amputation – she was not fit for a thoracotomy. They inserted a gastrostomy tube for feeding. I went to visit her on the ward for 'technical things', 'checking up' that she had good care plan, etc. I was really going there to be supportive. It should have been a two-minute visit but it wasn't. I went in there. I asked myself the cue, 'How must she be feeling?'. I pulled up a chair and asked her. She talked about vomiting."

CJ: "The ward staff had been dealing with this?"

Helen: "Yes but not appropriately. She was encouraged by our talk and then I asked how she was feeling. She just cried and cried and cried. She then apologised for crying, saying it would have been better not to have survived it at all. She talked of her feelings of loss – eating/independence/ her leg – her total feelings of being dependent. I let her talk about those things. I had just to be there for her – out it all came. She became calm again, began to talk about possible futures – talking about her leg rather than her stump. It felt really good to spend time with her in that way – almost nothing to do with her tube. That was just the by-line."

I challenged Helen: "It's got everything to do with her tube."

Helen was uncertain about this. I put the tube into perspective of the whole person: "You could only know her by seeing the tube?"

Helen accepted this perspective: "I felt overwhelmed, humble to get a sense of what she has lost. She doesn't have a lot of family. My next challenge is to go to the nurses and talk about how we are going to deal with it."

CJ: "You mean in terms of rehabilitation – her future?"

Helen: "Up to now she has been too sick. She is also isolated with MRSA in a sideroom. People spend as little time as possible with her because of that."

CJ: "The leper colony mentality."

Helen: "She would have been on the MRSA isolation ward if they had a bed."

CJ: "The paradox – someone who needs a lot of time to talk gets very little."

Helen: "Yes, have you heard the 'pizza jokes' about that – sliding them under the door so staff don't have to go in there."

CJ: "Did you confront that?"

Helen: "No, I am going back there today to follow it up. I want to talk to Vera, the ward sister, about it."

CJ: "Did you feel angry with the nurses?"

Helen: "Initially. I can see it exactly as it happens. They would say something like, 'It's all right for you swanning about all day. We're getting the job done'."

CJ: "You were angry for a short time and then you rationalised it?"

Helen: "It's not their fault. They were generally ignorant of the issues. My anger would have been a waste of time, it would have achieved very little. It happens everywhere. I want to use this anger positively rather than chew myself up."

CJ: "Can you use your anger positively?"

Helen: "By confronting people."

CJ: "You have been going around with this anger in you?"

Helen: "I think I am. I said to Melanie [colleague] 'Sometimes I really love my job. I am doing a good job, exciting and then something happens which makes me feel totally demotivated, upset, angry and like a very small cog in a very large wheel that doesn't 'give a monkey's' about me at all. How I seem to have been going round in this circle for years. I need to break out of this circle."

CJ: "Your task is to be assertive and feel yourself as a powerful person. Consider the way you manage conflict using the conflict management style grid (Box 7.4)"

Helen felt she was becoming increasing assertive yet was conscious of needing to establish collaborative relationships with ward nurses in order to do her job. Hence she had to tread a fine line, so perhaps compromise? With doctors Helen felt she had been accommodating because she needed to be accepted and valued by them.

Box 7.4 Thomas & Kilmann's (1974) two-dimensional model of conflict management (Cavanagh, 1991).

Assertiveness = the degree to which individuals satisfy their own concerns
Co-operation = the degree to which individuals attemp to satisfy the concerns of others

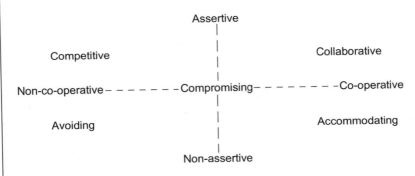

Accommodating
Essentially a co-operative interaction but one in which the practitioner is not assertive prepared to give up her own needs for the sake of maintaining harmonious relationships and need to be accepted by others. 'Apologetic.'

Avoiding
Characterised by a negation of the issues and a rationalisation that attempts to challenge the behaviour of another are futile.

Collaboration
Involves an effort to solve problems to a mutually satisfying conclusion – a win–win situation, i.e. concerned with needs of self and others. Openly discusses issues surrounding conflict and attempts to find suitable means to resolve the conflict.

Competitive
Pursues own needs at the exclusion of others, usually through open confrontation (win–lose situations).

Compromising
Realising that in conflict situations, every party cannot be satisfied. Accepts, at times, the requirement to set aside personal needs in order to resolve conflict.

CJ: "You need to reflect on the future for this woman -and what action you might take and what outcomes you would like."

Helen: "She is one of those women who has a real spark in her – intelligent, lively, funny – got it all there but needs help to get her out of this. She's had no rehabilitation for her leg as yet. I am not going to drop it!"

Being available

Helen highlighted her caring response to a distressed elderly woman and the way her motivation to confront her colleagues was fuelled by understanding the patient's feelings and her concern for the woman. She converted her 'outrage' into positive energy to take appropriate ation. The conflict management grid illustrates the way extant theory can be converted into a mapping technique. The grid was used over time to help Helen plot the development of her desired collaborative management style.

REFLECTIVE EXEMPLAR 7.5: THOMAS

At our next session Helen noted:

"I felt better about the limits of my responsibility by making the nurses on the ward aware. I tried to focus on my role responsibility and the relationship between seeing the tube and seeing the whole person, seeing the tube as part of the whole person, but I did feel I was getting into a mess. I can link this with a subsequent experience with Thomas."

Helen read from her diary: "Thomas has pancreatitis. He's very sick. He was having TPN through a Hickman line. I knew him from 10 years ago when he had cardiac problems. He latched on to me as 'his nurse', off-loading anxieties onto me. My visit to the ward was apparently routine to monitor the technology."

CJ: "What do you mean, 'apparently routine'? Has this changed?"

Helen: "This has changed already. It now includes 'Who is this person?' listening to the person, 'What is he asking/not asking me?' and it includes knowing 'How is this person feeling?' and 'How does he view the future?'. His pain was not being adequately dealt with. He was also frustrated at sitting and waiting for something to happen – that's the nature of his treatment. He was on a diamorphine pump for the pain – the technological response. Yet he was uncomfortable and unable to rest well enough. He was angry with the nurses about their handling skills. He felt they yanked him about. He was also frustrated at the nurses' comments and platitudes towards him.

I tried to help him consider less technological approaches to his pain management but he reacted against these. He had been socialised into technological responses and so he couldn't easily see beyond these. He was also venting his frustration at me. I didn't feel rejected. I went to see the ward staff. They were irritated at my interruption as they were trying to finish handover – trying to 'hurry up'. I had a sense of them being upset about something else. I acknowledged this feeling. They acknowledged that the ward was heavy at the moment, their own distress – lots of young patients with cancer and in particular a young girl who had been sexually abused by her father."

CJ: "In other words the staff were not available to you to talk about Thomas?"

Helen: "I sympathised with them but asserted I was trying to help them make it easier for themselves in nursing Thomas, who was already seen as a difficult patient."

CJ: "Are you always sensitive to their concerns?"

Helen: "Not always. I'm trying to be – they were obviously concerned about something that day."

CJ: "Were they surprised?"

Helen: "Yes, and pleased they had the opportunity to offload a bit. I responded by helping them talk through feelings concerning the sexually abused girl being discharged into the abused environment. They were distressed and felt helpless about this and other ways to help the girl."

CJ: "This is an example of how we have to deal with 'what's on top' before we can deal with our own agendas, otherwise the staff nurses may have simply rejected you and Thomas. To them, his needs were not as significant as this girl's."

Helen: "Most resistance to my ideas about Thomas came from the most newly qualified."

CJ: "Were you surprised by that?"

Helen: "You're going to tell me that I should have expected that!"

CJ: "Perhaps ... being least qualified she is unlikely to have the experience to fall back on and therefore she is more likely to see things as technical problems to solve and adopts technical decision-making processes. You exposed her technological response – that she was missing the point entirely."

Helen: "She used his 'anxious' disposition to account for his pain! She said things like, 'He's always asleep when you go in so I don't see how he can be in pain', all the kinds of things Thomas had been telling me about that irritate him so much!"

CJ: "So what happened?"

Helen: "I discussed other ways of dealing with his pain, although I didn't go far enough, such as suggesting pain charts. Afterwards I thought I should have done that. I was feeling irritated with them. I responded by telling them that they could avoid unnecessary complaint but perhaps this was not the best way to do this."

CJ: "I suppose you even quoted McCaffery (1983) to them? About pain being what the patient says it is."

Helen: "Funny enough I did! The staff nurse knew this quote but I don't think she believed in it."

CJ: "It exposes contradiction between theories we hold and how we practise. That was the confession bit from you – 'feeling irritated'. Is this uncomfortable for you?"

Helen: "Not uncomfortable – but knowing the best way of dealing with it."

CJ: "I think your intervention was valid. You were responding to help them see the consequences of not listening to you or Thomas."

Helen: "I wrote his kardex as a narrative and told the staff I had done that."

CJ: "What is the relationship between pain and TPN? Is pain management a legitimate concern of yours?"

Helen viewed Thomas within a holistic perspective where pain could not be separated from the whole. He was anxious about pain and this affected his acceptance of TPN. Therefore it was a legitimate part of her role.

CJ: "Why not send a copy of your new philosophy to each ward to help them *see* where you are coming from to legitimise your holistic approach. After all, he is your patient – they referred him to you!"

We explored the possibility of involving the named nurse in writing the notes during Helen's visit, highlighting a number of advantages:

- Legitimates Helen's role – involving staff explicitly means they negotiate – confronts people with their responsibility.
- Reinforces the named nurse concept on the ward.
- Teaches the named nurse, fulfilling teaching and supportive role.
- Develops relationships with the named nurses.
- Makes continuity of action more likely, therefore leads to better care.
- Breaks down ownership of the patient, leading to more mutual decision making that would help to reduce any conflict over authority for decision making.

I noted how Helen had managed her irritation in this situation, the way she monitored her feelings and contemplated other ways of responding. I suggested that she was irritated on two levels: first, because they were not accepting her expert advice and second, because she had taken on board Thomas's frustration and projected this frustration towards the nurses as though she were a mother whose child was hurt. Helen felt the first level was appropriate but hadn't perceived the second level until I drew her attention to this possibility.

Being available

Helen monitored and managed her anger towards the ward nurses. She tuned into the nurses' concerns and established a dialogue with them about responding appropriately to Thomas. In this sense she trod a fine line between asserting herself and Thomas's needs and marginalising herself as interfering, in which case Thomas's perspective and needs might not be readily acknowledged. Acknowledging the nurses' concerns made it easier for her to confront their unacceptable attitude and actions towards Thomas.

Helen was uncertain about her role boundaries and her legitimate authority for decision making. Her holistic perspective had shifted her boundaries – she was no longer just the 'tube lady'. However, shifting boundaries risked conflict with others who see the world differently and whose interests lie elsewhere, especially when the feedback is likely to expose poor practice.

REFLECTIVE EXEMPLAR 7.6: CATHY'S STORY

The therapeutic team requires colleagues to be open and assertive with each other, respecting and supporting the contribution each has to offer in the collaborative response to patients' needs. Cathy is a district nurse team leader and practice teacher. She uses the Burford NDU model to guide her work. Her story is concerned with a single experience she shared in her guided reflection with me over two sessions. Cathy talked about Brenda, an 84-year-old terminally ill woman she had been visiting each week since last summer.

Cathy: "I knew her from before when her husband had been ill. He had died. Brenda has had stomach cancer for which she had massive surgery. She had initially made a good recovery but then had a blockage which resulted in a stent being inserted. She was a deeply religious lady. Three weeks ago I was talking with her ... she seemed a little bit 'lost' – something about her. I was saying to myself, 'I'm sure next week you won't be here'. I couldn't put my finger on it ... perhaps the up before the major down. We were chatting about things we normally talk about. I said something like, 'See you next week Brenda'. She put a hand on my shoulder and said just as I was leaving, 'Yes, if God's willing' ... she gave me that look. She died later that week after being admitted to hospital."
CJ: "Were there other signs you could pick up?"
Cathy: "She was more relaxed ... she had talked about two of her friends who had died recently. She was quite a brave lady ... she didn't like tablets and she had pain in her back. We had tried different pain killers that had hardly touched her. I did notice that the lines she had around her eyes had gone ... her eyes looked bright, I thought."

CJ: "Intuitively you knew what she was saying to you – that she knew she was dying. Could you have responded differently at the moment?"
Cathy: "I didn't because I didn't know what to say . . . I had a cry in the car for her."
CJ: "She was saying good-bye. I suspect she didn't want any fuss about that. Did you go to her funeral?"
Cathy: "No . . . other things that needed to be done."

Cathy cried. I picked up on her tears and suggested that perhaps these were the tears she might have shed at the funeral. I named the various emotions she felt at this time: guilt at failing Brenda and her family, anger at the GP for admitting her to hospital, sadness at Brenda's death, anger at her own failure to act with integrity. A cocktail of energy-sapping emotions.

To deal with these I helped Cathy visualise a 'space' between us where she could 'dump' these feelings in order to view and understand them for what they were, to transform them into positive energy and to live with them more comfortably. I emphasised to Cathy that my role was not to fix it but to be there for her, role modelling how she might have been with Brenda if she had picked up that cue. I posed the question, 'How important is closing?'. Cathy had said before how important closing was. Cathy hadn't attended the funeral because of a management meeting she was expected to attend. I challenged her, 'Could you have prioritised differently? Could you have said to the GPs "Can you please reschedule this meeting so I can attend the funeral"? Would the GPs have understood your reasons for attending Brenda's funeral?'

Challenges for Cathy. Cathy said she now felt much better about the situation. In the session notes I raised two further challenges.

(1) Issue concerning where Brenda wanted to die, perhaps at home or a hospice rather than being admitted to hospital. Could this have been planned with her?
(2) Did you not pick up this cue because you wanted to avoid uncomfortable feelings because you felt so close to her?

In our next session three weeks later I drew Cathy's attention to the notes.

CJ: "Did you miss the opportunity for helping Brenda manage her death appropriately?"
Cathy: "Brenda definitely didn't want to go into the hospice. Her husband had died there. We had discussed this. She said, 'The hospice is a lovely place but I don't want to go into there because it brings back such memories'. She wanted to die at home . . . she had a strong family/friend network around her."
CJ: "What were the conditions of her readmission?"

Cathy: "The GP was a bit vague. He admitted her on the grounds of a range of deteriorating symptoms ... breathlessness. I was thinking of what you had said about the 'gap' on the Burford model study day about accepting the inevitable as inevitable ... and that the GP felt obliged to arrange her admission for treatment."

The 'gap' exists when there is a mismatch of expectation in managing the treatment trajectory. I had pictured a 'gap' between the nursing and medical time courses, where views did not coincide, a gap that represented the potential for conflict and breakdown of relationships.

```
                     Accept death as inevitable → focus on caring
Nursing  _____ |_____

                          Accept death as inevitable  → focus on caring
Medicine _____ |_____
              | Gap = potential for
                    conflict/breakdown |
```

Cathy could literally see this 'gap'. She had acknowledged the inevitability of Brenda's death before the medical team. She intuitively knew this and felt her appropriate response was to help Brenda die in comfort. The GP also intuitively knew the inevitability of Brenda's death yet within the unfolding moment could not accept this 'failure'. In response to her symptoms, he admitted her to hospital for treatment rather than arranging appropriate management of Brenda's death at home. The result was that Brenda was inappropriately admitted to hospital and died having to endure further painful treatment away from her home.

CJ: "Other ways of dealing with this?"

Cathy: "She was a strong character but she would have complied with what the GP said."

CJ: "It might be useful to debrief this situation with the GPs. Perhaps you could have insisted on being called if things deteriorated and you could have managed her at home. Issues of communication as well? I know in the emotional moment it was tough for you to respond to the cue she gave you, but we can see how circumstances unfolded that were not in her best interests, not in your best interests and an expensive alternative for the GPs – all issues about being proactive."

Cathy: "We are commencing a new series of meetings on Monday to improve communication! The idea is to have 'team care plans' where everybody knows what everybody else is doing."

Picking up the issue of priorities, funeral versus GP meeting, Cathy saw the funeral as a 'first' priority. She said: "In future I would be assertive about going to the funeral and say I would come to the meeting afterwards."

CJ: "Closing seems such important work. Can you find some literature to confirm that? I would like to know any literature on it. Knowing the 'evidence' may also help you in asserting your priorities with the GPs – 'the rational mind'. How might the GPs respond if you were to inform them that you weren't coming to their meeting but going to a funeral?"

Using the 'ethical map'

Cathy explored her dilemma within the 'ethical map' (see Box 7.5). Cathy identified and reflected on the different perspectives of those involved within the situation to understand the interplay of values and perceived authority that influenced how the decision was actually made. I acted out the part of the GPs, being scornful of Cathy's emotional responses and reminding her of her responsibility to the team. Cathy found it tough to assert her position. We then explored ways in which she could manage the situation: claiming the moral high ground, confronting their insensitivity without undue threat and giving them feedback on the significance of closing. I suggested that perhaps it might be best to pick the GPs off individually as together they have to perform to impress their colleagues.

Box 7.5 The ethical grid considering Cathy's dilemma.

Patient's/family's perspective: informs them that Cathy cared and is available to support the caring.	AUTHORITY TO ACT? Does Cathy have the autonomy to legitimately make this decision?	The doctor's perspective: going to the funeral is not the priority.
CONFLICT OF VALUES? Do Cathy and the GPs share a value system?	**Should Cathy be assertive about going to the funeral?**	ETHICAL PRINCIPLES? What is the greatest good? What is Cathy's greater responsibility?
The nurse's perspective: Cathy feels this is a greater priority than the meeting. Yet is this reasonable?	POWER RELATIONSHIPS? Why does Cathy go to the meeting?	The organisation's perspective: keep the GPs happy as they buy our services?

Influencing factors

Cathy then explored the factors that influenced her actions using the grid for considering the reflection cue, 'What factors influenced my actions?' (Boxes 7.6 and 7.7).

Box 7.6   Grid for considering 'What factors influenced my actions?' (Johns, 1998c).

My own expectations about how I should act?	Negative attitude towards the patient/family?	Expectations from others to act in certain ways? Conforming to normal practice?
Emotional entanglement?	**What factors influenced my actions?**	Misplaced concern? Loyalty to staff versus loyalty to patient/family?
Limited skills/discomfort in acting in other ways?	Time/priorities?	Anxiety about ensuing conflict? Fear of sanction?

Box 7.7   What factors influenced Cathy's actions?

My own expectations about how I should act?	Experienced as contradiction and inner conflict
Negative attitude towards the patient/family?	Cathy didn't feel negative towards the patient or the relatives. Indeed, she might have been accused of being too emotionally involved which blurred her perception of what's best.
Limited skills/discomfort in acting in other ways?	Cathy's discomfort prevented her from responding to the cue. However, she lacked confidence in cathartic and confrontational skills. Cathy perceived herself as non-assertive.
Time/priorities?	Cathy's Trust had significantly reduced the number of G-grade staff, forcing her into a team leader role to manage junior staff that had reduced her direct care contact. Hence, managing priorities had become a significant dilemma for her.
Expectations from others to act in certain ways? Conforming to normal practice?	GPs expected Cathy to attend the management meeting.
Misplaced concern? Loyalty to staff versus loyalty to patient/family?	Cathy felt forced to be loyal to her GP colleagues rather than Brenda and her family.
Anxiety about ensuing conflict? Fear of sanction?	Cathy was anxious to avoid conflict and sanction.

Being available

Cathy felt she needed to attend the funeral to close her relationship with Brenda and support Brenda's family. She felt she had failed Brenda, which distressed her. She did not attend the funeral because the GPs expected her to attend the meeting. Cathy had internalised this expectation as her own. She prioritised attending the meeting despite knowing this was not in her or Brenda's best interests.

Cathy's authority to act reflected the way she perceived power relationships. She perceived that she didn't have the authority to resist this expectation and anticipated conflict with the GPs if she did.

Cathy acknowledged that she was not assertive and had internalised a sense of the subordinate and powerless self *vis-à-vis* the GPs. This was evident throughout her experiences. However, she had worked hard at shifting this sense of self in order to feel more powerful within her caring values and to explore tactics to confront the GPs with their attitudes yet without marginalising herself. This is a fine balance. It is taking the moral high ground by presenting a coherent argument grounded in the patients' and relatives' interests and drawing on relevant research findings to confront the GPs with their own caring values. It would also lessen the risk that Cathy could be rejected as being emotional.

The shades of conflict within Cathy's story can be summarised in relation to different levels of managing conflict associated with levels of knowing (Box 7.8). Each level of conflict has to be resolved before the next can be dealt with adequately.

Box 7.8   Levels of conflict within practice.

Levels of knowing	Level of conflict	Cathy's experience
Knowing self	Intrapersonal	Cathy's unresolved distress (concern) about her own father's death that interferes with patients who are dying. Cathy tended to absorb the suffering of these patients and become entangled although this was not experienced as conflict.
Knowing therapeutic work	Interpersonal	Cathy avoided dealing with these feelings with Brenda, which possibly led to her admission to hospital.
Knowing responsibility and knowing others	Interpersonal	Cathy avoided asserting her caring beliefs in favour of the doctors' agenda.

Professional domination

Cathy's difficulty in asserting herself with the GPs can be understood within an underlying culture of patriarchy. One discourse of power relationships is to view nursing and caring as feminine against a dominant patriarchal view of medicine and managerialism. Watson (1990) has noted the barrier that patriarchy presents to the realisation of a caring society:

> 'Caring as a core value cannot be forthcoming until we uncover the broader more fundamental politic of the male-oriented worldview at work in our lives and the lives of people we serve.' (p. 62)

To help Cathy see herself in relation to the GPs, I guided her to explore relevant literature on the way nurses have struggled as a subordinate workforce in the face of medical domination (Hughes, 1971; Hughes, 1988; Kalisch, 1975; Capra, 1982; Clifford, 1985; Brunning & Huffington, 1985; Webster, 1985; Keddy *et al.*, 1986). Reverby (1987) explored how caring has been viewed as an extension of being a woman; indeed, as a woman's *duty* in contrast to her *work*. She asserted that this lack of power was largely a result of the relationship between womanhood and caring and the subordinate relationship of nurses to doctors where traditionally caring has been interpreted as the obligation to carry out the doctor's orders, an obligation that deprived nurses of rights. The effect of this history is a struggle to assert these rights even when nurses have a vision of caring as work.

Buckenham & McGrath (1983) highlight the way nurses have been socialised into passive, subordinate and powerless roles *vis-à-vis* medicine, which leaves them unable to fulfil their self-perceived role of patient advocate. They noted the way practitioners rationalised compliance with medical domination because of the need to be valued. It is natural for dominant professions such as medicine to reinforce subordinate behaviour in less dominant professions, such as nursing (Oakley, 1984).

Chapman (1983) suggested that doctors reinforced nurses' subordination through humiliation techniques which became a normal way of relating between them. Cathy felt coerced to submit to the doctors' view irrespective of what she felt was best. Although Cathy professed strong caring values, these values were not well articulated. Failure to articulate and assert caring values was disempowering. This is an important issue because patriarchy manifests itself in what counts as valid knowledge.

Lawler (1991) and James (1989) have both noted how caring in nursing was largely invisible, devalued by nurses themselves and seen as largely unskilled, being the natural extension of women's roles. Lawler's research was concerned with body work, whilst James was concerned with emotional work. Reflection enables practitioners to value caring as a significant aspect of practice. Reverby (1987) asserted that the real issues for nurses are caring and the conditions in which caring can be a reality rather than professional concern with autonomy which blurs the nursing purpose. Cathy's experience exposes the naivety of this position, demonstrating that practitioners need to be able to *assert* caring.

Perhaps there is a natural tendency to fall in with the beliefs wielded by social influence for the sake of harmony even when this is detrimental to one's own interests (Dewey, 1933). Dewey believed that shifting norms would disrupt normal working relationships and practices, highlighting how norms serve a social purpose in regulating what is accepted as normal practice. Action outside these norms is at once labelled as deviant and likely to result in conflict and sanctions to restore order.

Becoming assertive

Cathy, like many practitioners, was unable to be assertive with the GPs with whom she worked. She needed to learn to assert herself without margin-alising herself. In other words, the effective practitioner weighs her response to maximise its impact, yet also realising that within 'the corridors of power', the nursing voice is often unheard or easily dismissed as insignificant. Nurses may feel that they are not valued and that nursing has no say in health-care agendas. They may feel subordinate to doctors and managers and powerless to influence events, feelings reinforced daily through 'normal' ways of relating. The outcome of these norms is potential intrapersonal and inter-personal conflict as nurses are unable or unwilling to assert caring beliefs.

To help Cathy to develop her assertiveness, we focused first on under-standing the conditions which constrained her ability to assert her position. Second, we rehearsed assertive ways of responding whilst anticipating future situations. Third, we drew on reflective frameworks such as the assertiveness stereotype map (Box 7.9) and the asserting rights scale (Box 7.10) developed from the work of Dickson (1982), to help Cathy reflect on herself as asser-tive. Cathy used these maps through successive guided reflection sessions to plot the growth of her assertive self. With the GPs, Cathy felt she was Dulcie,

Box 7.9 Assertiveness stereotype map. Who do I best fit? (from Dickson, 1982)

	Dulcie (the doormat)	
	Selma (the assertive person)	
Agnes (the directly aggressive person)		Ivy (the indirectly aggressive person)

Box 7.10   Asserting rights scale (from Dickson, 1982).

(1)	I have the right to state my own needs and set my own priorities as a person independent of any roles that I may assume in life.
(2)	I have the right to be treated with respect as an intelligent, capable and equal human being.
(3)	I have the right to express my feelings.
(4)	I have the right to express my opinions and values.
(5)	I have the right to say 'yes' or 'no' for myself.
(6)	I have the right to make mistakes.
(7)	I have the right to change my mind.
(8)	I have the right to say I don't understand.
(9)	I have the right to ask for what I want.
(10)	I have the right to decline responsibility for other people.
(11)	I have the right to deal with others without being dependent on them for approval.

easily trodden on, and didn't score highly with asserting her rights. Using the maps is a visually empowering process.

A model of assertiveness

The practitioner's ability to be assertive hinges on a number of factors.

- A sense of the powerful self (the empowered self).
- Having a focused and strong vision of practice (the ethic to assert self).
- Understanding the boundaries of autonomy and authority in role (the right to assert self).
- Being able to make a 'good argument' (the knowledge to assert self).
- Being adept at interaction skills, most notably confrontational, cathartic and catalytic skills (Heron, 1975) (the skill to assert self).
- Being adept at counter coercive tactics against more powerful others (the resolve to assert self).
- Being able to manage defensive responses and conflict that may emerge in order to remain available within the moment (the managed self).
- Being able to 'tread the *fine line*' of confrontation without becoming marginalised and subsequently ineffective (the controlled self).
- Being able to create the optimum conditions to maximise the effectiveness of assertiveness, for example time of day, emotional climate, place, etc.

Towards collaboration

Asserting self may prompt a defensive or competitive reaction, especially from more powerful others who have traditionally responded to nurses as subordinates. The refusal to be passive and succumb to professional domination may provoke conflict and outrage that had previously simmered below the surface. Pike (1991) considered that the 'solution' to 'moral outrage' was the development of collaborative relationships between nurses and doctors based on a realisation of mutual trust.

However, collaboration is an ideal construct. Bishop & Scudder (1987) believe nurses need to focus on developing collaborative teamwork within the context of striving to achieve excellent practice. This is in contrast with a focus on individual autonomy as advocated by Yarling & McElmurray (1986). Bishop & Scudder noted that collaborative teamwork was difficult to achieve when members were concerned with their own autonomy, which would only lead to conflict within the system. Collaborative teamwork may be difficult to achieve unless both persons within the conflict are comfortable with their own sense of autonomy and respect that of others. Indeed, moral outrage is a reflection of the fact that collaboration between nurses and between nurses and doctors rarely exists within practice.

The rhetoric of collaborative teamwork may actually be unhelpful because it forces health-care workers to act as if this teamwork really exists, which makes conflict difficult to expose and resolve (Johns, 1996b). Bishop & Scudder's argument rests on an illusion that practitioners could be equal partners within decision making, an illusion which is not evident even between nurse colleagues, let alone with doctors and managers.

REFLECTIVE EXEMPLAR 7.7: MIRANDA'S RELATIONSHIP WITH LINDA

Miranda is a team leader working on an elderly care ward that used the Burford model. Her experience with Linda, her newly appointed manager, offers a view on the difficulty of shifting from hierarchical to collaborative relationships between nurses and managers.

> *Miranda*: "I had been away for 10 days and was trying to get back in tune with my patients – talking to them and reading through the notes. Linda came into the office. I immediately felt uncomfortable. I judged that she did as well – she made a light comment."
>
> *CJ*: "Jokey – taking the edge off things?"
>
> *Miranda*: "Yes, and then she withdrew and came along again when Tom [another team leader] was there and said to both of us that she wanted to have staff meetings to discuss practice with a view to changing things. I again felt very prickly. I felt two emotions, 'That's nice, but what does she want?'. She said, 'I need your support for changes, etc.' I was aware of my double reaction to her. I still feel the same way as it was occurring. I don't know whether she had the same feelings, perhaps we will have a chance to

talk about that. I did ask her how she was settling in. She said, 'I'm still learning the ropes – you probably know how I am feeling'."

Commentary

Miranda felt ambivalent towards Linda. On the one hand, she needed to be valued and on the other Linda threatened her autonomy. Miranda suggested that she expected Linda to adopt controlling behaviour, reflecting a deeply embodied sense of hierarchy.

In her next guided reflection session, Miranda read from her diary.

"Before going to work I felt nervous because I knew Linda had been working on the ward that morning. I sensed my standards were under observation. Before handing over we sat and talked about general issues. She said, 'I'll hand over first before going round. There's no particular order for doing things, is there?' I said that generally we walked round first to allow patients controlled disclosure, so that our observations and interactions weren't clouded by prior discussions between staff. She seemed genuinely surprised but accepted and walked round. I felt pleased to tell her that and expound the value of patient-controlled handover – teaching her something!

After the walk-round, she continued the handover in the office. I noticed she had developed good relationships with some of my patients. She seemed to be making a point of following planned care; she said, 'I did all I could after reading the care plans and notes'. She commented on some of the patients. I felt gratified that she had taken time in working with my patients and followed planned care, building relationships and being sensitive to the existing nurse–patient relationships. Prior to the handover I had felt concerned that she might find my care planning inadequate or inappropriate – I still have some uncertainty, even though I know I respond appropriately to patient-centred issues.

I know I was defensive, 'ready' for criticism although I couldn't be sure of what I was feeling and perhaps she was on the defensive herself or trying to develop trust between us before risking early criticism and even more defensiveness. Why *do* I feel insecure about my skills when she's giving care to my patients? I felt as if she made me feel inadequate and that I needed to justify all my decisions to her."

Commentary

Miranda's insight was revealing – that her confidence had evaporated with the threat of hierarchical control and judgement. She feared her work would become visible and found lacking. Miranda responded as a child expecting to be told off. Her fear of being exposed reflects a culture of traditional supervision, to ensure a competent and docile workforce whereby workers have internalised self-regulation (Foucault, 1979).

In the next session Miranda noted how helpful it had been to discuss her relationship with Linda last session: 'We talked openly about our situation even though I felt nervous. We shared our mutual expectations of roles which gave Linda the opportunity to talk about her fears of feeling "on trial". Rehearsal in supervision helped me to deal with that.'

Yet, in a later session seven months later, Miranda shared her reluctance about the proposed group supervision guided by Linda.

Miranda: "I would rather continue to have an external supervisor. I would be uncomfortable with my manager being the group supervisor."
CJ: "Do you know why you are uncomfortable with this idea?"
Miranda: "Because she is the senior nurse."
CJ: "Isn't that a contradiction if you believe relationships between staff should be collegial? Are you seeing her in an overt hierarchical relationship rather than collegial?"
Miranda: "It's a nice idea but difficult to achieve..."

Miranda talked through a number of difficulties within their relationship that had made her angry and which were unresolved.

CJ: "You are building up a picture of growing conflict between yourself and your manager ... can you take effective action?"

We explored Miranda's options and the consequences of these; for example, arranging individual supervision with her manager rather than with me.

CJ: "We have been talking about your manager as some third party – you need to talk to her directly and use supervision as a medium to establish a collegial relationship."

Miranda still felt her 'autonomy' was threatened by Linda. I could only respond by helping Miranda focus on positive action. Most significant would be to move into a supervision relationship with Linda and work towards developing a collaborative relationship congruent with team nursing (Manthey, 1980).

In the next session Miranda shared that she had been to see her manager and talked through a range of issues that had emerged from last session. Miranda noted that the meeting had been uncomfortable but had agreed to go into individual supervision as the means of resolving their conflict. They agreed to do some collaborative work on discharge evaluation.

Commentary

An advantage of line management guided reflection is the facilitation of collaborative relationships (see Box 3.8). Miranda's experience reflects that many practitioners have a deep distrust of management. This poses a dilemma: should Miranda accept being supervised with Linda in the knowledge that this relationship would create an opportunity to develop collaboratively? Or should Miranda choose who her supervisor might be? I believe that the onus is on the manager to deconstruct hierarchy rather than on the practitioner. Deconstructing hierarchy requires a letting go of positional power and a greater reliance on facilitative types of power (see Box 7.3) in working with each other towards mutual realisation of a shared vision. That is the essence of a reflective and holistic model for nursing.

Waterbutt theory of stress

The practitioners' stories reflect the significance of creating an environment that supports caring and dealing with factors that diminsh the practitioner's ability to care. The aim of support is to drain off negative energy and free energy for caring. The 'waterbutt' theory of stress management suggests that stress drip, drip, drips into self like a waterbutt slowly filling up. It is barely discernible until it reaches a level when it impairs being available. But by then it is too late to manage. It threatens to drown the person and all she can do is 'blow her top' to lower the stress. Sometimes the butt fills up very quickly, especially when the practitioner feels a sense of moral outrage at events and other people (Pike, 1991), is distressed (Wilkinson, 1988) or damaged (Parker, 1990). Pike noted:

> 'Moral outrage ensues when the nurse's attempts to operationalise a choice are thwarted by constraints. The outrage intensifies when these constraints not only block actions, but also force a course of action that violates the nurse's moral tenets.' (p. 351)

'Blowing her top' leaves an emotional mess which others anxiously mop up. No-one likes to see the outpouring of emotions, especially in a culture of the 'harmonious team'. Working with patients and colleagues is often stressful for whatever reason. Practitioners need colleagues to be sensitive and open to each other in the caring quest. By being self-aware, the practitioner can monitor the stress level within her 'waterbutt', draining it off appropriately and using this energy positively to resolve the issues that create stress, just as the gardener drains water from the butt to nourish plants. However, as the quote by Pike suggests, practitioners may need guidance to ensure the drainage tap is not blocked. This is the job of guided reflection or clinical supervision.

Burnout – the failure to sustain caring

Failure to achieve desirable work or manage anxiety in constructive ways may result in burnout. Cherniss (1980) described burnout as a process in which: 'The professional's attitudes and behaviour change in negative ways in response to job strain' (p. 5). Maslach (1976) suggested that the major negative change in those experiencing burnout in people-centred work was the: 'loss of concern for the client and a tendency to treat clients in a detached, mechanical fashion' (p. 6).

McNeeley (1983) observed that when practitioners felt they had lost the intrinsic satisfaction of caring, they became focused on the conditions of work, for example off-duty rosters and workload issues, characteristics of bureaucratic models of organisation. McNeeley believed that bureaucratic conditions were antithetical to human service work and strongly advocated that such organisations needed to move to collegial ways of working with staff to offset the risks of burnout. Taylor (1992) noted a theme within the literature of how nurses have been dispossessed: 'of their essential humanness as human beings and people, by emphasising their professional roles and responsibilities' (p. 1042).

Taylor draws attention to the fact that nurses are human too and as such are vulnerable to the same issues as their patients and families. The lack of recognition of humanness within nursing through a focus on roles and responsibilities led practitioners to strive to be something they clearly were struggling to cope with. Taylor noted that practitioners didn't recognise or understand their own ordinariness as human beings (p. 1044). Consequently, they became alienated from themselves in their efforts to cope with and live out the contradictions within their lives. Jourard (1971) noted that such striving damages 'the self' and reinforces the need to cope in a vicious downward cycle of self-destruction towards burnout and a state of anomie. Being patient centred may just perpetuate a denial of self that merely reinforces contradiction and is ultimately self-destructive. As Jade said, she didn't come to work dressed in protective armour. Dewey (1933) observed:

> 'Unconscious fears also drive us into purely defensive attitudes that operate like coats of armour – not only to shut out new conceptions but even to prevent us from making new observations.' (p. 30)

Dewey believed that anxiety limited the practitioner's ability to learn through experience. 'Armour' is akin to professional detachment. Benner & Wrubel (1989) believe that the answer is not the development of an adequate professional detachment, as advocated by Menzies-Lyth (1988), but the reconnection of the self with caring.

Clearly, burnout is not congruent with human caring. Yet are stress and burnout visible beneath the myth that good nurses cope? Nicklin (1987) noted that 85% of managers considered stress as only a moderate problem which they had no specific policy to deal with. The Briggs Report (DHSS, 1972) identified that services supporting nurses are rare, inadequate, fragmented and not targeted to those most in need. There is no evidence to suggest this situation has improved since 1972. In fact, the situation may have deteriorated due to the persistent asset stripping of nursing resources since the development of the business culture prompted by NHS Trusts. To say the least, it is ironic that a caring service should care so little about those who care. The emergence of clinical supervision is an acknowledgement of the need for formal support structures and the failure of informal support. However, clinical supervision is no substitute for the therapeutic team.

Chapter 8
Reflective Communication

Introduction

Communication ensures that care is continuous, consistent and congruent within and across practice settings. Communication can be through language, either verbal or written or non-verbal, through the body's posture and senses.

Consider each of your senses: smell, hearing (especially non-language), touch, sight. What do they communicate to you? The body is a reflection of the whole person, informing you of your inner self, whether you are open or defensive, anxious, introvert, angry. When next with a patient or family member, ask yourself what is being communicated in non-verbal ways. Do you pick up and respond to these cues? Next time in handover, pay attention to the non-verbal communication between staff. What is being said? What impact does it have?

Traditionally, nursing has relied heavily on an oral culture, exemplified by the handover. Handover is generally perceived as the handing over of responsibility of care from one nurse/one team of nurses to another nurse/ team by giving information. Perhaps an oral culture has diminished the significance of written notes to communicate patient and family care. Consider whether the patients' written notes in your practice adequately reflect the patient's care experience.

The nursing process

Since the late 1970s, the approach to patient care has been structured through the nursing process, a linear progression characterised by four stages.

(1) Goal setting – an interpretation of assessment to focus intervention on either actual or potential specific problems.
(2) Planning – establishing the best response to meeting the goals.
(3) Intervention – carrying out the planned care.
(4) Evaluation – determining whether the goal has been met, including redefining the problem or goal as necessary in light of events.

Each stage is written on the care plan. In theory, a practitioner should be able to pick up the care plan and continue to nurse the patient in a way consistent with previous care. However, most aspects of care cannot be prescribed in advance, at least not without reducing the human encounter to the status of an object to be manipulated. Some aspects of care may be more amenable to prescription – for example, technical solutions to medical problems such as wound dressings and responses to symptoms such as pain and nausea. These technical issues can be framed within protocols that guide the practitioner's best response in terms of evidence.

Beyond the nursing process

Although the nursing process was intended to promote a culture of individualised and negotiated care (De La Cuesta, 1983), ironically the opposite tended to happen when it was accommodated within a prevailing reductionist and deterministic culture of nursing practice. Rather than change practice, the nursing process has been accommodated to fit in within existing practice, resulting in minimal facilitation of individualised care (Latimer, 1995). Indeed, within a largely oral culture (Street, 1992), the requirement to process written notes became an irritation. Ineffective communication systems cease to function in any meaningful way. As such, written notes are neglected and do not reflect the care the patient needed, reinforcing the perception that the notes are indeed an ineffective method of ensuring the continuity of care.

The logic of the nursing process is grounded in a deterministic medical model legacy that a problem can be identified or 'diagnosed' and then the appropriate solutions can be applied to solve the problem. 'Problems' are seen largely as medically related physical problems in various systems or activities of living. Within the nursing process, 'planning' guides the practitioner towards a stereotyped perception of the patient as an object to be manipulated towards achieving certain predetermined outcomes. The mechanical nature of this process fits well with the way models of nursing have been conceptualised as reductionist: reducing the person to the status of a patient subsequently reducing the patient into systems or parts, essentially viewing the person as an object to be 'repaired' according to some rule book. From this perspective the nurse becomes a 'technician', fitting the person to the model.

This approach to planning care is blatantly deterministic. Determinism can only work at the level of technical response when the 'human factor' can be removed from the equation. In other words, the technical approach works in terms of manipulating an object towards a series of goals written in the care plan. The shadow of the medical model clouds a nursing perspective, adding a different level of determinism in that the problems identified on care plans are largely of a medical and physical orientation. The nursing diagnosis movement cultivated in the USA reflects a concern to shift this level of determinism towards a greater nursing orientation, albeit still at a level of imposing labels on both practitioners and patients.

From a holistic perspective, encompassing the self on a spiritual, emotional, psychological or social level, each caring encounter is unique between two human beings. It is an event that has never taken place before. Of course, this is why problems of a 'non-technical' nature seem so difficult to plan, often resulting in the practitioner using such stereotyped rhetoric as 'reducing anxiety' or 'reassure the patient' or interventions that are frankly insulting to the competent practitioner, such as 'enabling the patient to talk through her fears'. This level of planning suggests that practitioners are unable to consider such responses without triggers. Yet, when such issues are not written down they become invisible and are perhaps not reinforced as significant, in comparison with those care needs which are identified.

The inadequacy of the nursing process in guiding patient care means that practitioners do not use it. In an observational study of the impact of primary nursing on the culture of a community hospital (Johns, 1989), practitioners commented, 'Much of it is just nursing, you don't have to write that down, do you?' (p. 48) and 'Patients we know well don't need care planning' (p. 9). I asked one staff nurse on her return from her holiday if she had read the care plan. She commented, 'I haven't had time because it's so busy' (p. 45). One frustrated primary nurse commented, 'When I deliberately change something on the care plan, I came back from my days off and it hasn't been carried out ... is it because they disagree with what's been said or they are too busy to read the care plans? Not everyone will read the care plan and do as it says' (p. 46).

Updating the care plan becomes a retrospective *task* to be done at the end of the shift, reinforcing the notion that completing the notes lacks any utility value and meaning. Practitioners recognise this task as meaningless and yet are often anxious to write something, motivated by an internalised fear that if nothing is written then this may prove that care has not been given. The fear becomes reinforced when audit systems are constructed around the adequate completion of patient notes. Hence, what is written is itself descriptive and meaningless in terms of communicating the essential nature of continuing care.

The nursing process has attracted much adverse comment (Howse & Bailey, 1992; White, 1993; McElroy *et al.*, 1995; Latimer, 1995). If the nursing process is largely meaningless then, as Batehup & Evans (1992) have challenged, 'Why do we keep this sacred cow?'. Practitioners know this, yet have been unable to move beyond this deeply embodied worldview because the nursing process dominates the way nurses conceptualise their practice. Even when practitioners acknowledge the absurdity of the nursing process they seem powerless to move to more meaningful and practical ways of written communication.

The nursing process is an inadequate form of expression for the reflective practitioner because it does not represent how the reflective and holistic practitioner views and responds to situations. The Dreyfus & Dreyfus model of skill acquisition suggests that linear models are helpful to the novice practitioner who may lack experience (Benner, 1984). However, with increasing expertise, practitioners tend to make decisions based on intuition, drawing on past experience. In other words, reflective practitioners do not conceptualise in a nursing process way, perhaps explaining why practitioners are deeply dissatisfied with the nursing process. As practitioners begin to respond within a holistic perspective, the nursing process becomes a contradiction, making no allowance for the holistic and intuitive processes that are acknowledged as significant in the way experts make decisions about complex caring situations (Cioffi, 1997).

Narrative

Assessment and evaluation are two sides of the same coin – what is happening now and what has taken place before. The reflective practitioner is constantly processing this information in order to respond appropriately. The reflective practitioner has broken free of meaningless practice. Every action is both meaningful and pragmatic.

With these new sacred cows in mind, the reflective practitioner has no choice but to seek alternatives to the nursing process in writing and communicating about patient care. At Burford, practitioners moved to a narrative form that reflected the lived experience of working with the patient/family and other health-care workers. The narrative is a structured critical reflection that integrates assessment, evaluation, planning and intervention within the unfolding clinical situation. In other words, the narrative reflects the way the practitioner sequentially assesses the situation and evaluates what has gone before. She notes what was significant within the unfolding situation and what actions she has taken as a consequence. In continuing care the practitioner evaluates the efficacy of these actions in enabling the patient and family to meet their health needs.

Subnarratives

Within the traditional care plan at Burford hospital, evaluation was separated from care plans. The method was to number each problem on the care plan and then use that number to relate the progress notes to the problem. Consequently, when the practitioner was writing the progress notes she constantly needed to look back at the care plan and check through the notes to plot the history of the 'problem'.

Logically, the evaluation/progress notes need to be clearly linked to the care plan to ensure easy reference to the particular problem/health need. The narrative can be constructed as a series of subnarratives focusing on particular aspects of care. The change process involves taking people on a journey from familiar territory with a guide to show them the new scenery from a safe place at a safe pace. The shift from care plan to narrative can be summarised (Box 8.1).

Box 8.1   The culture shift from care plan to accommodate narrative.

Nursing process care plan	Reflective narrative
Admission focused – often the initial care plan sets the pattern of care without adequate continuous assessment	Assessment or pattern appraisal is a continuous process in which significant issues are constantly interpreted, negotiated and evaluated
Focus on problem or need – both actual and potential	Focus on problem or need – both actual and potential
Practitioner identification of a goal – often stereotyped	A shift from practitioners setting goals to patients and families being enabled to negotiate process and outcomes of care
Evaluation tends to be descriptive	Evaluation is reflective focusing on the significance of events
Mindset that something always needs to be written to prove that something has been done, usually as a task at the end of the shift	The practitioner only writes what is meaningful and practical
Culture of oral tradition and dissemination of information at handover	Shifting culture to emphasise written communication and reflective handovers

Structuring the narrative

The structure of the narrative is guided by the reflective cues (Box 2.2). Remember these are just cues, not concrete questions requiring concrete answers; they aim to trigger awareness of self with other within the particular moment, allowing the practitioner to pay attention to significant issues and the caring process.

The cues draw the practitioner into reflection, 'Who is this person?', at once acknowledging the person and countering the medical insidiousness of reducing the person to a patient. 'Who is this person?' not 'What is this disease, what are its symptoms, how is it investigated and treated?'. So how might the practitioner write about 'Who is this person?'? The reflective accounts throughout the book tell the story ... read again my accounts of being with Tony. See the way their stories unfold and what is significant within them.

My response to Tony, as with all people, is an interpretation of finding meaning, yet a meaning focused on the person's particular experience rather than my own experience of similar situations. As such, I pay attention to 'who I am' within this process, checking myself constantly for the interpretations I am making, not drawing hasty conclusions based on my accumulated knowing in practice. Central to this interpretative process is the knowledge that the person is here with me for a reason that is generally determined by a health crisis or, in midwifery and health visiting, by normal health events. The midwife and health visitor are companions to inform and ease the way.

Contemplating the cue 'How do I feel about this person?'

I have often been asked, 'How does the practitioner write in the notes about her response to the reflective cue "How do I feel about this person?"'. First, the practitioner needs to remember that this is a 'cue' – it tunes the practitioner into her own feelings and concerns that may interfere with being available to the patient/family. If the feeling is negative then the practitioner needs to consider how to respond to her own 'concerns' in therapeutic ways. If the negative feeling is triggered by something about the patient/family's behaviour, then the best way is to acknowledge this difficulty using a cathartic-type response – 'I can see you are anxious'. This is also cathartic for the practitioner as she responds to her own anxiety in understanding the significance of the event and cautions her against absorbing the patient's anxiety as her own.

The nurse might write something like: 'Sheila is very anxious. I acknowledged her anxiety and enabled her to surface and talk through her fears … [list]'. Her emotional reaction might be: 'Sheila's anxiety manifests itself as *demanding and abusive*'. The practitioner may have initially felt abused and defensive but she does not write it. In other words the practitioner writes about what she has done with her concern rather than about the concern itself. She has acknowledged the patient's feeling as valid and converted her own anxiety into positive action, acknowledging that the patient and her family may be bewildered and overwhelmed by events and possibly even angry at the way things have unfolded, especially when the patient's life is at risk or when other health-care workers have lacked concern.

The nurse manages this interface between the patient/family and the organisation. She can be a soft target to fire at. And yet the reflective practitioner senses the tension. She gently exposes and confronts it, in order to respond appropriately. The skilled practitioner can learn to manage her own concerns in order to be available. She knows that the patient's behaviour is usually a manifestation of the health event and not antisocial behaviour *per se*, although it might eventually require confrontation. Clearly, if the patient/

family have the opportunity to read their own notes, then these notes cannot be antagonistic.

REFLECTIVE EXEMPLAR 8.1: REG SIMPSON

Consider the way the reflective cues structure Reg Simpson's narrative.

Admitted this morning from home for one week's respite care, Reg has been attending day care [see attached notes]. Reg is 93. He suffers from carcinoma of the prostate gland. He lives alone. His two daughters live close by and provide support for him. However, as Reg says, he is not managing so well. This morning he was in a real mess getting dressed, feels he will need more support. His daughter needed a break from caring, hence this admission.

Reg wears a hearing aid, requires fairly loud voice to hear. He is very philosophical about this admission and indeed, about his eventual death. He was tearful when talking about his wife who died 27 years ago. I asked him if he anticipated being reunited with her. He laughed and said no. He had no strong belief – he thought he would just return to the earth from whence he came. He enjoys the *Guardian* newspaper, doing crosswords and watching TV. Very keen angler but fears he may lose this – so dependent on help to go fishing. He enjoyed chatting – was very appreciative of this chat with him, especially talking about philosophical issues.

Reg presents with a number of care issues.

(1) Anxious about his sleep. He commenced sleeping tablets six weeks ago. These have been helping. He was waking up at 4 AM and becoming distressed as he lay awake for remaining five hours until he got up. He goes to bed around 10–10.30 PM.
Action – monitor sleep
(2) No complaints of pain or other disease-related symptoms.
(3) He has a number of other medical problems, treated with a range of drugs [see list] – not an issue for him. He has tubigrip to both lower legs – some oedema evident.
(4) Poor appetite and loss of taste. He enjoys soups. He says he has significant weight loss. However, he takes this issue in his stride.
(5) Increased loss of mobility. He has given up using his electric scooter at home – he was getting his feet mixed up! Walks with a zimmer, in fact walked with one nurse to eat lunch at table. No confidence.
Action – review by physiotherapist
(6) Fragile skin: he has small break on hand – accident with his grandson. No other breaks. Will need pressure relief equipment [see Waterlow/lifting-handling assessment].
Action – monitor pressure areas: Wound is 2 cm × 1 cm stage 2. Dress daily with non-adhesive allevyn and secure with bandage

(7) He has a catheter *in situ* – he doesn't like it but it is working okay.
(8) He says he is prone to constipation – I didn't ask when he last opened his bowels.
     Action – monitor
(9) Support for the future
     Action – to discuss with daughters current situation/to support his daughters

He is likely to require assistance with washing/ dressing tomorrow.
He said he enjoyed his soup for lunch. Even managed some pudding!

Day 2

New wound noted on outer side of right leg. Size 1 cm × 4 cm. Stage 2. Treat daily with adhesive allevyn. He knocked his leg on the side of the bed. Current pressure area caution is adequate. He has been seen by physiotherapist – see her notes. He can walk with zimmer and one nurse safely. He really enjoyed his 'jacuzzi' bath this morning.

Sleep – use sleep visual analogue scale. Reg woke again at 4 AM and lay restless until breakfast. We need to review our approach as it distresses him.

Medication (currently temazepam 10 mg).

This afternoon he was dozing in chair, he says he does this at home. He asked me the time. I said 4 PM – he groaned 'Oh no – when is dinner time?'. Clearly bored, he structures day through meal events. I asked him how the crossword went yesterday. He said he hadn't been in the mood. I found him the *Telegraph* for today – Hazel said she would help him do it later. He enjoys company.

Reg seen by Dr Webb – he is booked for thyroid function test on Monday. Also to review the prolonged use of sertaline – antidepressant. Does he need this?

Day 3

Sleep – pattern of waking at 4 AM continued. Using the sleep visual analogue scale [VAS] – he was not satisfied. Explore alternatives to increased temazepam?

Introduced bowel chart – as no action. No complaint from him. Like his sleep problem, he is resigned to these niggling problems. Spent time with him doing the crossword before he dozed off for much of the afternoon – perhaps this is why he struggles with his sleep later.

Day 4

VAS repeated – no shift in pattern. Wounds observed after bath – healing satisfactorily. We talked again about his future and support. He is conscious of being a burden though says his daughter is very caring. He accepts his forthcoming death with no regrets. Good chat.

Daughter visited – she feels able to manage both physically and emotionally. Thankful for respite care. No significant anxiety about supporting Reg although she doesn't talk with him about dying. I fedback his attitude – she says 'I know he's okay about it but I still find it difficult'. I gave her a hug and asked what she would like to do about this. It's okay for the moment but she felt pleased to know she can contact me as necessary or Louise in day care. Some tears.

She's going away for a few days – will pick him up from day care next Monday afternoon. Contact number on front sheet.

Commentary

There is no prescription as to the best way to write a narrative. Remember the maxim – be meaningful and practical. However, it is not easy to shift from previous ways of conceptualising and writing about practice. It may initially help to use the reflective cues in a more deliberate way. Slowly the cues are internalised, enabling the practitioner to stop thinking consciously about them, yet still structuring the response to the person and family.

Contemplating the cue, 'What support does this person have in life?'

Reg's notes reflect the dialogue between the practitioner and Reg's daughter, checking out how she is feeling and managing with Reg's care at home. Does she need additional support, how does she view the future for Reg and for herself? Reg was a respite care patient which often means that our contact with the family is minimal because the idea is to give the family a break from caring.

Self-assessment

Self-assessment creates the opportunity for the practitioner to get certain information from the family prior to or at the point of admission, especially if the person being admitted is a poor historian. It is not easy for the carer to hand over care to another. Dawson (1987) noted that spouses in particular equate caring duty with marital responsibility, leading to a strong sense of guilt when the spouse requires admission for respite care. Does this tell the world the spouse has failed and can no longer manage? The carer may experience anxiety that hospital carers cannot know the patient well enough or feel they have lost control of the caring role. I am sure all nurses know of the interfering spouse who complains bitterly that the patient is not receiving good enough care. This is the spouse's anxiety being projected onto the caring staff. The reflective practitioner reads this pattern and enables the spouse to surface and work through the anxiety.

Self-assessment may provide a way for the carer to:

- set out in detail the patient's normal lifestyle;
- feel in control and involved in the care process;
- feel recognised and valued as the main carer;
- have his or her own needs recognised as a legitimate focus for care.

The self-assessment form devised at Burford had ten sections. The first nine sections focused on identifying patient's needs.

(1)   Personal hygiene needs
(2)   Dressing needs
(3)   Eating and drinking needs
(4)   Toilet needs
(5)   Mobility needs
(6)   Sleep needs
(7)   Daily activity and communication needs
(8)   Psychological needs
(9)   Anything else to make the patient's stay in hospital comfortable

Section 10 focused on the carer's needs. Box 8.2 illustrates a wife's assessment of her needs related to caring for her husband who was terminally ill with bowel cancer. The wife presented a brave face of caring but actually was at the end of her tether. Using the form was cathartic and enabled her to disclose in a way she had difficulty doing verbally, opening the way for her needs to be recognised and acknowledged as valid and to get much needed support.

The carer's assessment becomes the basis for negotiating care on admission. All the 'little things' that are important for the patient's care have been identified and acknowledged to minimise the risk of the patient's and carer's normal routines and lifestyle being disrupted. Hopefully, the carer can then enjoy her or his break in a more relaxed frame of mind.

Mapping

In constructing a sub-narrative, scales, charts, graphs and maps offer a visual way to *scan* the pattern of care.

Sleep visual analogue scale (VAS)

The sleep VAS (Box 8.3) offers a way for the patient to monitor her own satisfaction with sleep. Sleep is an important aspect of living that may easily get overlooked as a significant caring factor. The work of Martha Rogers (see Chapter 1) has drawn attention to the interconnection between self and environment. Consider the significance of sleep for yourself, especially when

Box 8.2   Self assessment for carer needs.

How are you generally coping with the person at home?	*Reasonably well but there is no let-up . I am 77 years old.*
Do you have any particular problems or area of concern with caring?	*No, only cleaning up accidents – not so bad latterly.*
What support are you receiving at home? Is this support adequate?	*I have a certain amount of help with cleaning – nurse to bath my patient weekly – hopefully help from Social Services to help him wash and dress – this in the pipeline.*
Are you able to identify any further support you might need?	*Not as yet, must see how the above works.*
How do you anticipate the future?	*With trepidation, but I take each day as it comes.*
When did you last get a break from caring?	*Never, since the illness started, apart from laser beam treatment at the church.*
Do you get a break from care from other sources?	*No.*
Has it been necessary for you to care for a friend or relative previously?	*Only with my mother many years ago.*
How was that for you?	*Difficult because of my own family's needs.*
How does caring affect your usual pattern of living?	*One tends to drop out of local events because it is so time consuming and exhausting.*
How do you feel about your relative coming into hospital?	*Slightly apprehensive as he is a home bird but I know he will have every care possible.*

Box 8.3   Sleep visual analogue scale (VAS)

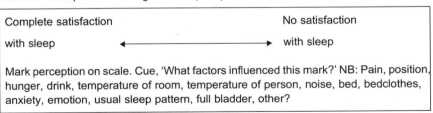

Complete satisfaction   No satisfaction

with sleep   ◄─────────────────► with sleep

Mark perception on scale. Cue, 'What factors influenced this mark?' NB: Pain, position, hunger, drink, temperature of room, temperature of person, noise, bed, bedclothes, anxiety, emotion, usual sleep pattern, full bladder, other?

you have been ill. As with other environmental factors such as eating and the physical environment, sleep may be a neglected aspect of caring practice – taken for granted in the technology-dominated environment.

The VAS comprises a 10 cm line along which the patient marks their satisfaction with sleep. The practitioner then enquires about the factors that the patient feels have interrupted her sleep. The chart may include a checklist of possible factors to trigger the patient's response: anxiety, comfort, pillows, position, usual life patterns such as time for going to bed and rising, lack of company, rituals such as prayer, drinks, reading, light, medications, getting up in the night for the toilet. Anxiety may be major factor that disrupts sleep. The reflective cue, 'What is important for this person to make their stay in hospital comfortable?' draws the practitioner's attention naturally to discuss these kinds of issues with the patient. Using the sleep VAS gives this attention a structure and a way to monitor and record whether sleep satisfaction has been achieved.

I used the sleep VAS to assess and monitor Reg's satisfaction with sleep. Monitoring the sleep VAS is illustrated with two patients – Mrs Duncan and Mrs Longworth.

Mrs Duncan

Complete satisfaction
with sleep

No satisfaction
at all with sleep

10   *   0

Baseline reading: score 1.5

Comment: Mrs Duncan identified that her poor satisfaction with sleep was due to her husband being very elderly and disturbing her. She continued to sleep with her husband. She had been transferred to Burford for rehabilitation following hernia repair surgery. Whilst at the general hospital she had been prescribed temazepam, one tablet at night. She brought these tablets with her.

Complete satisfaction
with sleep

No satisfaction
at all with sleep

10   *   0

First reading: score 8.5

Comment: Discussed with Mrs Duncan and the GP the need for temazepam. The GP discontinued it in order to wean her off it prior to discharge. Mrs Duncan said she felt okay about this.

Complete satisfaction
with sleep

No satisfaction
at all with sleep

10   *   0

Second reading: score 0.5

Comment: The second reading showed a dramatic reduction in her sleep satisfaction. When this score was discussed with her, she complained that her GP wouldn't let her have temazepam and that she had got herself into a state about it. In other words, Mrs Duncan had only superficially complied with the decision to stop the temazepam. The night staff reported Mrs Duncan had slept well, illustrating how deceptive observation of a person's sleep can be compared with the person's own subjective experience or what they might report when casually asked. The associate nurse discussed again with Mrs Duncan the problems associated with prolonged use of temazepam. The associate nurse suggested that Mrs Duncan could try to manage without them that night. Mrs Duncan agreed.

Complete satisfaction
with sleep
 No satisfaction
at all with sleep

10 *   0

Third reading: score 9.5

Comment: The next night, Mrs Duncan had almost complete satisfaction with sleep. She continued to sleep well for the rest of her stay in hospital. Talking through her anxiety and her control of the decision to stop the temazepam reassured her. The issue of being disturbed by her husband was not discussed with her. Her recognition that this was the cause of her poor sleep satisfaction at home may enable her to change this situation. With hindsight, she may have been helped to consider solutions to this problem.

Mrs Longworth

Complete satisfaction
with sleep
 No satisfaction
at all with sleep

10   *   0

Baseline reading: score 1.5

Comment: Mrs Longworth felt this score was due to her severe arthritic hip pain. She was waiting for a total hip replacement. To offset the pain she took Distalgesic which she self-administered. She was accustomed to sitting in a chair at home during the night.

Complete satisfaction
with sleep
 No satisfaction
at all with sleep

10   *   0

First reading: score 3.5

Comment: She had taken two Distalgesic last thing but had still been woken by pain. She was again woken by the nurses seeing to the lady in the next bed. She commented, 'They are very quiet really, I can't grumble'. Despite the low score she remarked, 'on the whole I'm quite satisfied'.

Complete satisfaction   **No satisfaction**
with sleep   **at all with sleep**

10   *   0

Second reading: score 1.0

Comment: Mrs Longworth had woken at 1 AM and described her pain as 'shocking'. She had taken two hours to get back to sleep. She remarked, 'I took more tablets which isn't usual for me'. She disclosed that at home she sat in the chair which she didn't do here because she didn't want to disturb the nurses. It was arranged for her to have an appropriate chair next to her bed the following night.

Complete satisfaction   **No satisfaction**
with sleep   **at all with sleep**

10   *   0

Third reading: score 6.0

Comment: Mrs Longworth said she felt much better. Clearly the pattern of her normal sleep habit should have been recognised earlier. Whilst her discomfort was eased I felt that her increased satisfaction was also due to the recognition of her normal lifestyle and management of this need. Trusting people with chronic illness to take control of aspects of their life in which they feel competent has been shown to be positively related to their satisfaction with health care (Thorne & Robinson, 1988).

The sleep VAS proved to be a useful tool to prompt practitioners to discuss with patients factors that influenced satisfaction with their sleep. Attention to such detail is a powerful caring phenomenon. As a consequence, practitioners became very sensitive to the sleep environment.

Bowel chart

While it feels almost heretical to suggest a return to the 'bowel chart', mapping is a practical and meaningful approach to monitoring the pattern of bowel action. At a glance, the pattern over time is revealed alongside the efficacy of response. This chart was designed at a hospice, where constipation is a particular problem for many people – patients, families and nurses! Before the introduction of the bowel chart, a standard care plan was used

Date	Shift am pm night	Open y/n	Assessment Description	Response *1 Evaluation

that stated a universal goal: 'The patient should have their bowel open 1–3 days (depending on what's normal for them).' The care plan also stated the universal initial response: 'one bisacodyl and one glycerine suppository'. Whilst this response may generally be the most appropriate, it may not be so for each patient. The risk in implementing this intervention is to stereotype the response to the problem. A better approach to the standard care plan is to construct a protocol for managing constipation.

Protocols

As the reader may have observed, the focus of experience throughout the book has been on relational rather than technical issues. This is not to say that technical issues of nursing practice are not significant. Clearly they are but they do not often present as problematic for practitioners within guided reflection. Where they are raised by practitioners, they are often presented as 'how' and 'why' type questions, as suggested by Van Manen (1977).

Managing aspects of care such as bowel care, pain management and wound care should be guided by 'evidence' based on current theory and research findings. Whilst protocols ensure safety and consistency of approach, it is important to emphasise that they merely inform the practitioner's judgement rather than being a prescription to reduce the person receiving care to an object to be manipulated towards specific outcomes.

Reflective handover

Given the general paucity of written notes, the verbal handover might be considered the most significant form of communication. To reinforce their value within everyday practice, written notes need to be actively utilised when handover of care between practitioners takes place. The practitioner can be asked to read from the notes. Alternatively, the practitioner might only highlight significant shifts in the patient's care trajectory or use the handover space to raise care issues for reflection, encouraging her colleagues to share opinions and feelings and talk over more difficult aspects of care. Such an approach shifts the culture of the handover from information dissemination to reflective debate. Of course, time is always at a premium, but the practitioner receiving handover can spend a few minutes reading the notes after the handover period. Indeed, incomplete information will prompt the nurse to acquaint herself more fully with the patient's care.

Traditionally handover is a verbal communication between the practitioner responsible for managing care and the practitioner accepting responsibility for continuing care. This often takes place in the staff office and excludes the patient. However, handover can also provide an opportunity to involve the patient as part of the ongoing existential dialogue. In such cases, the handover moves from the office into the patient care environment – described as the walkabout handover. Based on experience at Burford, I believe that handover is best commenced with the walkround to discuss with each patient's care with them. This is patient controlled prompted by the practitioners. The intention of this approach is to enable:

- the oncoming nurse to meet the person;
- the patient to be actively involved in his care and to give his perspective.

Staff must honour confidentiality by ensuring that information about the patient is not heard by others. A breach of confidence cannot be tolerated because it reflects an attitude of disrespect. As such, it is uncaring and creates anxiety and breakdown of trust. The patient may, of course, choose to disclose information.

Following the walkround, the handover can be continued in the office to 'fill in' gaps of information and continue the caring dialogue. The patient's narrative is explicitly used for this purpose. At Burford, patients were informed and asked to give their consent for communicating with and about them in this manner. If the patient felt uncomfortable about his involvement, this was respected and yet negotiated for its appropriateness. The patient may be resisting responsibility which may not necessarily be in his best interests. By reading the person's pattern the nurse can acknowledge and confront this response.

The way practitioners hand over care at Burford was written as a protocol (Box 8.4). The protocol is clearly influenced by the practitioner's beliefs about 'working with' the patient and family. Box 8.5 sets out the literature that was searched to inform our practice.

Managing quality

In Box 2.1 I set out an expanded view of a reflective model for nursing incorporating a system to ensure the model realises effective practice. To be

Box 8.4 Protocol for communication at han~~d~~
states that health care workers work with
meaning in the health care experience, to mak~~e~~
negotiate care. Handover between health care ~~staff~~
to be realised whilst respecting that some p~~atients~~
negotiating their care.

Stage	Action
1	The nurse who orientates the pers~~on~~ patient's attention to the style of con~~duct~~ (stated in the hospital's information~~) ~~ patient's right not to be involved in h~~ ~~ ....~~~~egotiated.
2	Handover time between day staff and night staff is at 20.45 and 08.00. Handover between day staff occurs at a mutually convenient time.
3	Handover *commences* with nurses visiting patient. The nurses may invite others as appropriate to join the handover. This approach is referred to as 'the walkround'. It enables the: • nurse to see/say hello to the patient; • nurses to involve the patient in negotiating care (as able and desired); • patient to give their perspective on caring first; • nurses to save time by avoiding repetition.
4	The patient's right to confidentiality during the handover as advised by the UKCC (1987) is respected. As such, nurses act to enable the patient to control the disclosure of information. The nurse handing over may sensitively cue the patient to prompt disclosure as appropriate.
5	Following 'the walkround', the nurses continue the handover in the staff room to 'fill in' gaps of information and understanding.
6	The primary means of continuing consistent care is through the use of patient narratives. These are actively used as the basis of communication between nurses.
7	Following the verbal handover, the nurse continuing care assures herself of patient need through continuing the patient's narrative. This necessitates the update of the narrative by the nurse handing over.
8	The patient's notes are clearly marked with the patient's name and stored by the patient's bed within the storage basket.

Box 8.5 Involving pat~~ients~~
Ashworth, P. D~~.~~
meaning~~ ~~
17: 14~~ ~~
Biley~~ ~~

consistent with reflective and holistic practice, such a system needs to be grounded in reflective and holistic technique. One way to get feedback of quality is through guided reflection. The practitioner reflects on the quality of care, enabling a judgement to be made as to whether the quality is adequate

...ents in decision making – literature sources.

..., Longmate, M. A. & Morrison, P. (1992) Patient participation: its ...and significance in the context of caring. *Journal of Advanced Nursing* ...30–9.
... F. C. (1992) Some determinants that affect patient participation in decision-making about nursing care. *Journal of Advanced Nursing* **17**: 414–21.
Butterworth, T. (1996) Individualised nursing care: a cuckoo in the team's nest? *NT Research* **1** (1): 34–7.
Gadow, S. (1980) Existential advocacy. In *Nursing: Images or Ideals?* (Spickler, S. and Gadow, S., eds). Springer, New York.
Jewell, S. E. (1994) Patient participation: what does it mean to nurses? *Journal of Advanced Nursing* **19**: 433–8.
Mallick, M. (1992) The role of the nurse on the consultant's ward round. *Nursing Times occasional paper* **89** (5): 49-52.
Matthews, A. (1986) Patient-centred handovers. *Nursing Times* **82** (24): 47–8.
McMahon, R. (1990) What are we saying? *Nursing Times* **86** (30): 38–40.
Morse, J. (1991) Negotiating commitment and involvement in the nurse–patient relationship. *Journal of Advanced Nursing* **16**: 455–68.
Redfearn, S. (1996) Individualised patient care: its meaning and practice in a general setting. *NT Research* **1** (1): 22–33.
Rowe, M. A. & Perry, M. (1984) Don't sit down nurse, it's time for report. *Nursing Times* **85** (26): 42–3.
Trnobranski, P. H. (1994) Nurse–patient negotiation: assumption or reality? *Journal of Advanced Nursing* **19**: 733–7.
Waterworth, S. & Luker, K. A. (1990) Reluctant collaborators: do patients want to be involved in decisions concerning care? *Journal of Advanced Nursing* **15**: 971–6.
Watkins, S. (1993) Bedside manners. *Nursing Times* **89** (29): 42–3.

Confidentiality
Johns, C. C. (1989) To whom it may concern. *Nursing Times* **85** (39): 60–1.
Newton, T. (1986); Protecting data. *Senior Nurse* **4** (3): 10–11.
UKCC (1987) Advisory paper: confidentiality – an elaboration of clause 9. UKCC, London.
Ward, K. (1988) Not just the patient in bed three. *Nursing Times* **84** (78): 39–40.

or not. The practitioner's performance can be systematically summarised in reflective reviews as part of a quality system (see p. 67). A more formal reflective way to manage quality is by constructing reflective standards of care (Johns, 1998d).

Standards of care

At Burford, we formed a reflective practice group that met monthly to reflect on and develop specific aspects of nursing practice. Each aspect of practice was written as a standard of care that reflects desirable practice. Standards can either be written on specific problems that practitioners become aware of or as a systematic attempt to address all areas of practice. For example, the handover protocol was written as part of a standard: 'Patients do not have confidential information disclosed about them accidentally'.

The need to write the standard emerged from observing poor practice during the walkabout handover when information about a patient was overheard by other patients in the shared ward area. I raised my concern with the practitioners involved and then suggested that the standards group reflected on how this aspect of practice could be improved. A standard concerned with patients' sleep was prompted by a complaint by a patient that she had not slept well during her stay at Burford. The sleep VAS was developed as a tool to monitor the ensuing standard: 'Usual sleep patterns are maintained to the patient's comfort'

In writing a standard the reflective group:

- brainstorm significant factors that seem pertinent around the particular aspect of practice by reflecting on specific situations;
- search the relevant literature to determine what might be construed as 'best practice'. For example, the literature reviewed for the handover protocol is shown in Box 8.5. This literature is stored in a resource file on patient involvement in decision making/handover – a useful resource for staff and students!
- consider the resources that are necessary to achieve the standard of practice (structure criteria). Standards of care must capture the tension between what is desirable and what is achievable in terms of resources. Resources are reviewed in order to maximise efficiency;
- consider the actions required of all practitioners and workers to achieve the standard of practice (process criteria). A protocol sets out the actions required by practitioners and as such, would be part of the process criteria within a standard of care;
- Consider ways in which the standard of practice can be monitored to ensure the desired standard is met (outcome criteria).

Monitoring

The most effective monitoring tools are based on either observation or asking the patient and family direct questions. The scan sheet for the standard, 'Patients do not have confidential information disclosed about them accidentally' is shown in Box 8.6. The scan sheet also includes a specific question to ask the patient. The practitioner monitoring the standard marks the extent to which she felt each criterion was met and notes situations when it wasn't met. She then feeds back to the staff involved and files the scan sheet in the standard file. As a rule of thumb, the more the standard is seen as not being met, the more frequently scans should be undertaken.

Box 8.6 Confidentiality standard scanning sheet.

	Max.	Min.
Patients do not have confidential information disclosed about them accidentally.		

Patients do not have confidential information disclosed about them accidentally.

Max.   Min.

(1) Patients are involved in the handover of
     their care   ─ ─ ─ ─ ─ ─ ─ ─ ─ ─ ─ ─ ─ ─ ─

(2) Patients control the disclosure of
     information concerning themselves   ─ ─ ─ ─ ─ ─ ─ ─ ─ ─ ─ ─ ─ ─ ─

(3) The nurses do not talk about the patient
     out of 'listening'   ─ ─ ─ ─ ─ ─ ─ ─ ─ ─ ─ ─ ─ ─ ─

(4) No accidental breach of confidentiality
     occurs   ─ ─ ─ ─ ─ ─ ─ ─ ─ ─ ─ ─ ─ ─ ─

(5) The nurses talk primarily with the patient   ─ ─ ─ ─ ─ ─ ─ ─ ─ ─ ─ ─ ─ ─ ─

(6) Are patients' notes left open in a public
     place?   ─ ─ ─ ─ ─ ─ ─ ─ ─ ─ ─ ─ ─ ─ ─

(7) Ask each patient, 'Do you think your nurses have always treated what they know
     about your health problems in a confidential manner?'

Sleep standard

The complete sleep standard is shown in Box 8.7, illustrating the way standards are reduced to specific structural, process and outcome criteria.

Writing standards sensitises practitioners to discrete aspects of care and consequently has a powerful impact on care. Monitoring standards becomes integral with caring itself. The benefits of writing reflective standards of care are summarised in Box 8.8.

Conclusion

The reflective approach outlined in this book is not prescriptive. There are no right answers, except to be open to new ideas which requires a constant challenge to review all ways of working for their appropriateness in tune with the unit philosophy. Change may prove difficult because organisations have often established computerised information and audit systems around documentation. Yet this fact should not obscure the fundamental issue that the nursing process is merely a tool to facilitate the communication of effective practice. If the tool is inappropriate then it should be discarded in favour of more meaningful and practical systems for communicating care. Does the expert carpenter choose a spoon to shape his wood? Clearly not. He chooses a sharp chisel which he uses to create the perfect joint. The expert practitioner

Box 8.7   Sleep standard (adapted from Burford standard, March 1989). Usual sleep patterns are maintained to the patient's comfort.

1.0   Structure criteria
1.1   Telephone in reception muted at night/staff to use telephone in casualty
1.2   Dimmer lights fitted and working to all beds
1.3   Patient call bell system volume reduced at night (agreed with engineer)
1.4   The patient can negotiate a change of bed position if desired (as posible)
1.5   The patient is able to bring his or her own bedlinen/pillow, etc. into hospital (as possible within fire regulations)
1.6   Sleep resource person/resource file on sleep in library

2.0   Process criteria
2.1   The nurse considers environment disruptions to patient's sleep and acts to minimise these (via VAS)
2.2   The nurse recognises and plans to meet the patient's usual pattern for daytime activity and sleep
2.3   The nurses act to minimise patient disturbance throughout the night

3.0   Outcome criteria

3.1   Factors that limit and enhance patient's satisfaction with sleep are adequately responded to (reflected in increased satisfaction with sleep – via VAS)

Box 8.8   Benefits of standards of care.

Standards of care offer the practitioner:

- a framework to develop all aspects of clinical practice;
- a dynamic 'bottom-up' change management model;
- a way of making a philosophy for practice a reality in practice;
- a process for group reflection and leaning through experience;
- a resource management model;
- a means for the practitioner(s) to demonstrate professional accountability by making quality part of everyday practice;
- the means to write nursing quality into business contracts;
- a quality assurance tool tailored to practice that captures the tension between desirable and achievable practice.

---

always chooses the most appropriate tools for the job. Of course, this argument applies to all aspects of care.

Nurses, midwives and health visitors everywhere seek to enable and care for people and families requiring some health-care intervention to have their needs met. They seek to work in collaborative ways with people and families, and with their colleagues. The stories and theories shared in the book illuminate the significance of reflective practice as a way of enabling practitioners to realise their caring destiny. Caring is not a passive process. It requires great commitment, compassion and expertise. It also requires perseverance and courage when working in environments that constrain the practitioner's ability to care in desirable and effective ways. Yet first, it requires a strong sense of vision to focus the caring effort, to draw practitioners together in common quest. I have suggested that caring requires reflective structures that facilitate caring in everyday practice alongside reflective developmental processes that are congruent with the clinical process. Reflection gives the practitioner access to self in context of her practice – to know, nurture, develop and sustain self as caring. Yet the profound nature of this work may require guidance to fulfil its developmental potential.

Reflection opens the doors of perception for practitioners to fulfil their caring destiny in ways that transform not just themselves but the whole of health care. Tuck this book under your arm as you proceed along your own caring and reflective journey as a guide along the way. Remember, the book does not set out to be prescriptive of what you should do but offers, through the multiple stories, experiences and their interpretations, a source of knowing for you, the reader, to relate to in terms of your own experiences. Good journeying!

Postscript
Jean Watson

And just what are we to make of becoming a reflective practitioner? Are we to learn? Are we to change? Are we to work toward transformation of self and other?

This work by Christopher Johns brings us face to face with the human elements and human dilemmas, the deep level of humanity that clinicians encounter daily, moment by moment, the blessings and challenges of living, suffering, changing, evolving, dying, leading us to nothing less than a rebirthing of self and work. And how are we to live this practice of reflection? How are we to be? To become? To evolve? To alter? To repattern? To rethink?

We do so by stepping into practice moments; we do so by honouring our own inner humanness; we do so by stopping, being present, listening to stories, life narratives, filled with inner meanings, myths, metaphors and inner soul lessons gleaned from the field, in the field. In seeking soul lessons, by reflecting on one's own presence of being and becoming in the moment. It is through the reflective moment that we both seek and gain insights, dynamics of wisdom and depth of meanings revealed whole to us but only when we stop, pause and are present to such profound human mystery and wisdom that is already contained on the margin, in the shadows, in the distant haze of our own existence.

It is here, when we are still, witness to our own openness, that we connect with self and other in shared moments of human being and becoming. A multifaceted jewel, the diamond net of refracted light contained within each moment of human encounter ... a clue, a coloured hue, contributing to a human canvas, a human studio of caring moments, each one a possibility for hope, for movement through pain, suffering, loss, challenge, while being present to the joy; the aesthetic, the paradox, the dilemma, the eternal, uncovered from the journey toward wholeness. In the nurse's presence, in listening to and becoming part of another's story, life drama, myth for meaning and hope, we are able to promote health or become true instruments of timeless healing that transcend self, other and system alike.

Reflective stories in this text offer models of insight; they reveal the hidden subtext of paradox, inner drama, unaddressed questions, unknowns, that lead to ethical grids and maps on the reflective journey – a reflective journey, into context, discovery, relationships, non-objectivist, non-formulaic notions and moods that guide not by convention and rationalistic principles but rather by intentional consciousness, by awakening. Awakening to presence, relationships, being and becoming part of the connections, patterns and processes that mirror human-to-human caring and healing.

This reflective subtext of nursing invites us into and through informed, reflective, appropriate skilled action of human connectivity, creativity and intuition. Through internal and external existential dialogue story and guidance we journey into the spiritual, the aesthetic, the ethical, the arts, that touch and celebrate the non-quantifiable, that once again reunite the profession and the practitioner alike, with the compassion and passion of nursing's life and work.

It is here through the Johns reflective practice model and its evolving process for self-reflection and guidance that we discover, once again, that the 'personal becomes the professional'. It is here that we learn to grow in caring by becoming instruments of healing, first by learning about our own inner healing and health processes and needs that flow from self to other. These lessons transcend yet inform each caring moment, consciously or unconsciously. It is through reflective practice that nurses and nursing learn about nursing as never known before. It is here, in honouring the whole, in gleaning and seeking meaning from parts and particles of light in the institutional and often individual darkness, that we find new hope for transforming nursing and nurses alike.

Finally, it is through reflective practice, as continually explored and explicated by Johns and colleagues, that we are offered a method, a mode, a mood, a model of being and becoming that allows us to face and live through, if not be blessed by, our own woundedness. This model is a guide that informs and invites us, in uniquely individual ways, to engage in authentic caring and become part of a process of healing and wholeness that is required for a new era in human history and futuristic nursing.

In the past nurses and nursing have tried to escape the inner learning and healing that is required for the practice journey; we have done this by succumbing to medical science, medical-nursing tasks, industrial-system demands. It has turned out that these routes to nursing have been a detour from our human caring practices and commitment to processes of wholeness and healing that have motivated, inspired and informed individuals and communities across time.

It is through the breakdowns of conventional practices, combined with breakthroughs of reflective practice, which can now be integrated with the most up-to-date knowledge and skills, philosophies and theories, that we enter a new world of professional care practices that embrace, encompass and more fully actualise the paradigm of hope spread before and behind nursing in its history and traditions. It is only by stopping, pausing and reconsidering our encounters and relationships with self and other that we mature as a distinct caring, healing and health profession.

However, it is the reflective practice processes and approaches that may be the most threatening, yet at the same time offer the greatest hope for growth, maturity and personal and professional maturity. If nursing turns its back on reflection, it is turning its back on its woundedness and core humanity, which is the ground of being and becoming. In not pausing to consider reflection, we remain technical assistants, trying to defend ourselves from our own wounds and suffering, forever stranded on the shoreline as humanity and health care itself sets out to pursue new horizons of possibilities contained within the depths of our shared humanity and the oceanic changes possible for human evolution and growth.

Will we choose reflection and human transformation as a path to the future or succumb to robotic mutation? Which route will we take? Reflect upon it and choose but do so with passion and purpose. As we individually and collectively ponder the future, this text offers a holistic lesson that will serve us well into the new millennium.

References

Alfano, G. (1971) Healing or caretaking – which will it be? *Nursing Clinics of North America* **6** (2): 273–80.

Allen, D. (1987) Critical social theory as a model for analysing ethical issues in family and community health. *Family and Community Health* **10** (1): 63–72.

Armitage, S. (1990) Research utilisation in practice. *Nurse Education Today* **10**: 10-15.

Atkins, S. & Murphy, C. (1993) Reflection: a review of the literature. *Journal of Advanced Nursing* **18** (8): 1188–92.

Atkinson, R. L, Atkinson, R. C. & Smith, E. E. (1990) *Introduction to Psychology.* Harcourt Brace, New York.

Bailey, R. & Clarke, M. (1989) *Stress and Coping in Nursing.* Chapman and Hall, London.

Batehup, L. & Evans, A. (1992) A new strategy. *Nursing Times* **88** (47): 40–1.

Barrett, E. (1990) Health patterning with clients in a private practice environment. In *Visions of Rogers' Science-Based Nursing* (Barrett, E., ed.), pp. 105–15. National League for Nursing, New York.

Belenky, M. F., Clinchy, B. M., Goldberger, N. R. & Tarule, J. M. (1986) *Women's Ways of Knowing: the Development of Self, Voice and Mind.* Basic Books, New York.

Benjamin, M. & Curtis, J. (1986) *Ethics in Nursing*, 2nd edn. Oxford University Press, New York.

Benner, P. (1984) *From Novice to Expert.* Addison-Wesley, Menlo Park.

Benner, P. & Wrubel, J. (1989) *The Primacy of Caring.* Addison-Wesley, Menlo Park.

Betz, M. & O'Connell, L. (1987) Primary nursing: panacea or problem? *Nursing and Health Care* **8**: 456–60.

Bishop, A. & Scudder, J. (1987) Nursing ethics in an age of controversy. *Advances in Nursing Science* **9** (3): 34–43.

Blackwolf Jones, R. & Jones, G. (Earth Dance Drum. Commune-A-Key Publishing, Salt Lake City.

Bohm, D. (1980) *Wholeness and the Implicate Order.* Routledge and Kegan Paul, London.

Bolen, J. S. (1996) *Close to the Bone: Life Threatening Illness and the Search for meaning.* Touchstone, New York.

Bond, M. & Holland, S. (1998) *Skills of Clinical Supervision for Nurses.* Open University Press, Buckingham.

Boud, D., Keogh, R. & Walker, D. (1985) Promoting reflection in learning: a model. In *Reflection: Turning Experience into Learning* (Boud, D., Keogh, R. & Walker, D., eds). Kogan Page, London.

Boyd, E. M. & Fales, A. W. (1983) Reflective learning: key to learning from experience. *Journal of Humanistic Psychology* **23** (2): 99–117.

Brookfield, S. (1987) *Developing Critical Thinkers*. Open University Press, Buckingham.

Brunning, H. & Huffington, C. (1985) Altered images. *Nursing Times* **81** (31): 24–7.

Buckenham, J. & McGrath, G. (1983) *The Social Reality of Nursing*. Adis, Sydney.

Burnard, P. & Morrison, P. (1991) Nurses' interpersonal skills: a study of nurses' perceptions. *Nurse Education Today* **11**: 24–9.

Callahan, S. (1988) The role of emotion in ethical decision making. *Hastings Center Report* **18**: 9–14.

Callanan, M. & Kelley, P. (1992) *Final Gifts*. Bantam Books, New York.

Capra, F. (1982) *The Turning Point: Science, Society and the Rising Culture*. Fontana, London.

Carmack, B. J. (1997) Balancing engagement and detachment in caregiving. *Image: Journal of Nursing Scholarship* **29** (2): 139–43.

Carper, B. A. (1978) Fundamental patterns of knowing in nursing. *Advances in Nursing Science* **1** (1): 13–23.

Carr, W. & Kemmis, S. (1986) *Becoming Critical*. The Falmer Press, Lewes.

Casement, P. (1985) *On Learning from the Patient*. Routledge, London.

Cavanagh, S. (1991) The conflict management style of staff nurses and managers. *Journal of Advanced Nursing* **16**: 1254–60.

Chapman, G. E. (1983) Ritual and rational action in hospitals. *Journal of Advanced Nursing* **8**: 13–20.

Cherniss, G. (1980) *Professional Burn-out in Human Service Organisations*. Praeger, New York.

Chopra, D. (1989) *Quantum Healing: Exploring the Frontiers of Mind/Body Medicine*. Bantam Books, New York.

Cioffi, J. (1997) Heuristics, servants to intuition, in clinical decision-making. *Journal of Advanced Nursing* **26**: 203–8.

Clifford, C. (1985) Conflict or co-operation. *Nursing Practice* **1** (2): 102–8.

Coleman, P. (1986) *Ageing and Reminiscence Processes: Social and Clinical Applications*. Wiley, Chichester.

Cooper, M. C. (1991) Principle-oriented ethics and the ethic of care: a creative tension. *Advances in Nursing Science* **14** (2): 22–31.

Cowling, W. R. III (1990) A template for unitary pattern-based nursing practice. In *Visions of Rogers' Science-Based Nursing* (Barrett, E., ed.), pp. 45–66. National League for Nursing., New York.

Cox, H. Hickson, P. & Taylor, B. (1991) Exploring reflection: knowing and constructing practice. In *Towards a Discipline of Nursing* (Gray, G. & Pratt, R., eds), pp. 373–90. Churchill Livingstone, Melbourne.

Cox, M. (1988) *Structuring the Therapeutic Process: Compromise with Chaos*. Jessica Kingsley Publishers, London.

Dawson, J. (1987) Evaluation of a community based night sitter service. In *Research in the Nursing Care of the Elderly* (Fielding, P., ed.), pp. 87–106. Wiley, Chichester.

Day, C. (1993) Reflection: a necessary but not sufficient condition for professional development. *British Educational Research Journal* **19** (1): 83–93.

De La Cuesta, C. (1983) The nursing process: from development to implementation. *Journal of Advanced Nursing* **8**: 365–71.

Department of Health and Social Security (1972) *Report of the Committee on Nursing* [Chairperson, Professor Asa Briggs]. HMSO. London.

Dewey, J. (1933) *How We Think*. J. C. Heath, Boston.

Dickson, A. (1982) *A Woman in Your Own Right*. Quartet Books, London.

Drew, N. (1986) Exclusion and confirmation: a phenomenolgy of patients' experience with caregivers. *Image: Journal of Nursing Scholarship* **18** (2): 39–43.

Dreyfus, H. L. & Dreyfus, S. E. (1986) *Mind Over Machine*. Free Press, New York.

Dunlop, M. J. (1986) Is a science of caring possible? *Journal of Advanced Nursing* **11**: 661–70.

Farrar, M. (1992) How much do they want to know. *Professional Nurse* **7** (9): 606–10.

Fay, B. (1987) *Critical Social Science*. Polity Press, Cambridge.

Ferrell, L. (1998) Doing the right thing: customary vs reflective morality in nursing practice. In *Transforming Nursing Through Reflective Practice* (Johns, C. & Freshwater, D, eds). Blackwell Science, Oxford.

Field, D. (1989) *Nursing the Dying*. Tavistock Routledge, London.

Fitzgerald, M. (1994) Theories of reflection for learning. In *Reflective Practice in Nursing* (Palmer, A., Burns, S. & Bulman, C., eds). Blackwell Science, Oxford.

Forrest, D. (1989) The experience of caring. *Journal of Advanced Nursing* **14**: 815–23.

Fossbinder, D. (1994) Patient perceptions of nursing care: an emerging theory of interpersonal competence. *Journal of Advanced Nursing* **20**: 1085–93.

Foucault, M. (1979) *Discipline and Punish: the Birth of the Prison* (trans. A. Sheridan). Vintage/Random House, New York.

Freire, P. (1972) *Pedagogy of the Oppressed*. Penguin Books, Harmondsworth.

French, J. R. P. & Raven, B. (1968) The bases of social power. In *Group Dynamics: Research and Theory*, 3rd edn (Cartwright, D. & Zander, A., eds). Harper and Row, New York.

Gadamer, H-G. (1975) *Truth and Method*. Seabury Press, New York.

Gadow, S. (1980) Existential advocacy. In *Nursing: Image and Ideals* (Spickler, S. & Gadow, S., eds), pp. 79–101. Springer, New York.

Gibbs, G. (1988) *Learning by Doing: a Guide to Teaching and Learning Methods*. Further Education Unit, Oxford Polytechnic, now Oxford Brookes University.

Greene, M. (1988) *The Dialectic of Freedom*. Teachers' College Press, Columbia University, New York.

Habermas, J. (1984) *Theory of Communicative Action. Vol. 1: Reason and the Rationalization of Society*. Beacon Press, Boston, and Basil Blackwell, Oxford, in association with Polity Press, Cambridge.

Hall, L. (1964) Nursing – what is it? *Canadian Nurse* **60** (2): 150–4.

Halldórsdóttir, S. (1996) Caring and uncaring encounters in nursing and health care–developing a theory. Linköping University Medical Dissertations No. 493. Linköping, Sweden.

Hardy, H. (1997) Learning to know self through guided reflection. A new study of caring for adolescents in hospital. Unpublished BA Health Care Studies dissertation, University of Luton.

Hawkins, P. & Shohet, R. (1989) *Supervision for the Helping Professions*. Open University Press, Buckingham.

Heron, J. (1975) *Six-Category Intervention Analysis*. Human Potential Resource Group, University of Surrey, Guildford.

Hingley, P. & Cooper, C. (1986) *Stress and the Nurse Manager*. Wiley, London.

Holly, M. L. (1989) Reflective writing and the spirit of inquiry. *Cambridge Journal of Education* **19** (1): 71–80.

Howse, E. & Bailey, J. (1992) Resistance to documentation – a nursing research issue. *International Journal of Nursing Studies* **29** (4): 371–80.

Hughes, C., Blackburn, F. & Walgo, M. (1986) On masking among clients. *Topics in Clinical Nursing* **3** (1): 83–9.

Hughes, D. (1988) When nurse knows best: some aspects of nurse/doctor interaction in a casualty department. *Sociology of Health and Illness* **10** (1): 1–22.

Hughes, E. C. (1971) *The Sociological Eye: Selected Papers*. Aldine-Atherton, Chicago.

Hunt, J. (1981) Indicators for nursing practice: the use of research findings. *Journal of Advanced Nursing* **6**: 189–94.

James, N. (1989) Emotional labour: skill and work in the social regulation of feelings. *Sociological Review* **37** (1): 15–42.

Johns, C. (1989) The impact of introducing primary nursing on the culture of a community hospital. Master of Nursing Dissertation, University of Wales College of Medicine.

Johns, C. (1992) Ownership and the harmonious team: barriers to developing the therapeutic nursing team in primary nursing. *Journal of Clinical Nursing* **1**: 89–94.

Johns, C. (1993) On becoming effective in taking effective action. *Journal of Clinical Nursing* **2**: 307–12.

Johns, C. (1994) *The Burford NDU Model: Caring in Practice*. Blackwell Science, Oxford.

Johns, C. (1995a) Time to care? Time for reflection. *International Journal of Nursing Practice* **1**: 37–42.

Johns, C. (1995b) Achieving effective work as a professional activity. In *Towards Advanced Nursing Practice* (Schober, J. E. & Hinchliff, S. M., eds), pp. 252–80. Edward Arnold, London.

Johns, C. (1995c) Framing learning through reflection within Carper's fundamental ways of knowing. *Journal of Advanced Nursing* **22**: 226–34.

Johns, C. (1996a) Visualizing and realizing caring in practice through guided reflection. *Journal of Advanced Nursing* **24**: 1135–43.

Johns, C. (1996b) Understanding and managing interpersonal conflict as a therapeutic nursing activity. *International Journal of Nursing Practice* **2**: 194–200.

Johns, C. (1997a) Reflective practice and clinical supervision. Part 2: Guiding learning through reflection to structure the supervision 'space'. *European Nurse* **2** (3): 192–204.

Johns, C. (1997b) Caitlin's story – realizing caring within everyday practice through guided reflection. *International Journal for Human Caring* **1** (2): 33–40.

Johns, C. (1998a) Becoming an effective practitioner through guided reflection. PhD thesis. Open University, Milton Keynes.

Johns, C. (1998b) Caring through a reflective lens: giving meaning to being a reflective practitioner. *Nursing Inquiry* **5**: 18–24.

Johns, C. (1998c) Opening the doors of perception. In *Transforming Nursing through Reflective Practice* (Johns, C. & Freshwater, D., eds), pp. 1–20. Blackwell Science, Oxford.

Johns, C. (1998d) Developing a reflective standard of care. *Nursing Times* **94** (8): 54–6.

Johns, C. (1999a) Unravelling the dilemmas within everyday nursing practice. *Nursing Ethics* **6** (4): 287–98.

Johns, C. (1999b) Caring connections; knowing self within caring relationships through reflection. *International Journal for Human Caring* 3 (2): 31–8.

Johns, C. (1999c) Reflection as empowerment? *Nursing Inquiry* (in press)

Johns, C. & Freshwater, D. (eds) (1998) *Transforming Nursing through Reflective Practice*. Blackwell Science, Oxford.

Johns, C. & Graham, J. (1996) Using a reflective model of nursing and guided reflection. *Nursing Standard* 11 (2): 34–8.

Johns, C. & Hardy, H. (1998) Voice as a metaphor for transformation through reflection. In *Transforming Nursing Through Reflective Practice* (Johns, C. & Freshwater, D., eds), pp. 51–61. Blackwell Science, Oxford.

Johns, C. & McCormack, B. (1998) Unfolding the conditions where the transformative potential of guided reflection (clinical supervision) might flourish or flounder. In *Transforming Nursing through Reflective Practice* (Johns, C. & Freshwater, D., eds), pp. 62–77. Blackwell Science, Oxford.

Johnson, D. (1974) Development of theory: a requisite for nursing as a primary health profession. *Nursing Research* 23 (5): 373–7.

Jourard, S. (1971) *The Transparent Self*. Van Nostrand, Norwalk, CT.

Kalisch, B. J. (1975) Of half-gods and mortals: aesculapian authority. *Nursing Outlook* 23 (1): 22.

Keddy, B., Gillis, M., Jacobs, P., *et al.* (1986) The doctor–nurse relationship: an historical perspective. *Journal of Advanced Nursing* 11: 745–53.

Kieffer, C. H. (1984) Citizen empowerment: a development perspective. *Prevention in Human Services* 84 (3): 9–36.

Kikuchi, J. F. (1992) Nursing questions that science cannot answer. In *Philosophic Inquiry in Nursing* (Kikuchi, J. F. & Simmons, H., eds). Sage, Newbury Park.

King, L. & Appleton, J. V. (1997) Intuition: a critical review of the research and rhetoric. *Journal of Advanced Nursing* 26: 194–202.

Knowles, M. S. (1980) *The Modern Practice of Adult Education*. Follet, Chicago.

Kramer, M. K. (1990) Holistic nursing: implications for knowledge development and utilisation. In *The Nursing Profession: Turning Points* (Chaska, N., ed.). C. V. Mosby, St Louis.

Kübler–Ross, E. (1969) *On Death and Dying*. Macmillan, New York.

Larson, P. J. (1987) Comparison of cancer patients' and professional nurses' perceptions of important nurse caring behaviours. *Heart and Lung* 16 (2): 187–93.

Latimer, J. (1995) The nursing process re-examined: enrolment and translation. *Journal of Advanced Nursing* 22: 213–20.

Lawler, J. (1991) *Behind the Screens: Nursing, Somology, and the Problems of the Body*. Churchill Livingstone, Melbourne.

Levine, S. (1986) *Who Dies? An Investigation of Conscious Living and Conscious Dying*. Gateway Books, Bath.

Lieberman, A. (1989) *Staff Development in Culture Building, Curriculum and Teaching: The Next 50 Years*. Teachers' College Press, Columbia University, New York.

Luft, J. (1970) *Group Processes: An Introduction to Group Dynamics*, 2nd edn. National Press, New York.

Luker, K. (1988) Do models work? *Nursing Times* 84 (5): 27–9.

Macleod, M. (1994) 'It's the little things that count': the hidden complexity of everyday clinical nursing practice. *Journal of Clinical Nursing* 3 (6): 361–8.

Madrid, M. (1990) The participating process of human field patterning in an acute-care environment. In *Visions of Rogers' Science-Based Nursing* (Barrett, E., ed.), pp. 93–104. National League for Nursing, New York.

Manthey, M. (1980) *The Practice of Primary Nursing*. Blackwell Scientific Publications, Boston.

Margolis, H. (1993) *Paradigm and Barriers: How Habits of Mind Govern Scientific Beliefs*. University of Chicago Press, Chicago.

Marris, P. (1986) *Loss and Change*. Routledge and Kegan Paul, London.

Marshall, J. (1980) Stress amongst nurses. In *White Collar and Professional Stress* (Cooper, G. L. & Marshall, J., eds). Wiley, Chichester.

Maslach, C. (1976) Burned-out. *Human Behaviour* **5**: 16–22.

May, C. (1991) Affective neutrality and involvement in nurse–patient relationships: perceptions of appropriate behaviour among nurses in acute medical and surgical wards. *Journal of Advanced Nursing* **16**: 552–8.

Mayer, D. K. (1986) Cancer patients' and families' perceptions of nurse caring behaviours. *Topics in Clinical Nursing* **8** (2): 30–6.

McCaffery, M. (1983) *Nursing the Patient in Pain*. Harper & Row, London.

McElroy, A., Corben, V. & McLeish, K. (1995) Developing care plan documentation: an action research project. *Journal of Nursing Management* **3**: 193–9.

McNeely, R. L. (1983) Organizational patterns and work satisfaction in a comprehensive human service agency: an empirical test. *Human Relations* **36** (10): 957–72.

McSherry, W. (1996) Raising the spirit. *Nursing Times* **92** (3): 48–9.

Meehan, T. C. (1990) The science of unitary human beings and theory-based practice: therapeutic touch. In *Visions of Rogers' Science-Based Nursing* (Barrett, E., ed.), pp. 67–82. National League for Nursing, New York.

Menzies-Lyth, I. (1988) A case study in the functioning of social systems as a defence against anxiety. In *Containing Anxiety in Institutions: Selected Essays*. Free Association Books, London.

Mezirow, J. (1981) A critical theory of adult learning and education. *Adult Education* **32** (1): 3–24.

Miller, H. (1939) *Tropic of Capricorn*. Flamingo, London.

Milne, A. A. (1926) *Winnie-the-Pooh*. Methuen, London.

Moore, T. (1992) *Care of the Soul*. Harper Collins, New York.

Morse, J. (1991) Negotiating commitment and involvement in the nurse–patient relationship. *Journal of Advanced Nursing* **16**: 455–68.

Morse, J., Bottorff, J., Meander, W. & Solberg, S. (1991) Comparative analysis of conceptualisations and theories of caring. *Image: Journal of Nursing Scholarship* **23** (2): 119–26.

Moss, R. (1981) *The I That is We*. Celestial Arts, Millbrae, CA.

Newell, M. (1992) Anxiety, accuracy, and reflection: the limits of professional development. *Journal of Advanced Nursing* **17**: 1326–33.

Newman, M. (1994) *Health as Expanded Consciousness*, 2nd edn. National League for Nursing, New York.

Nicklin, P. (1987) Violence to the spirit. *Senior Nurse* **6** (5): 10–12.

Noddings, N. (1984) *Caring – A Feminine Approach to Ethics and Moral Education*. University of California Press, Berkeley.

Nolan, M. & Grant, G. (1989) Addressing the needs of informal carers: a neglected area of nursing practice. *Journal of Advanced Nursing* **14**: 950–61.

Norbeck, J. (1985) Coping with stress in critical care settings: research findings. *Focus on Critical Care* **12**: 36.

Oakley, A. (1984) The importance of being a nurse. *Nursing Times* **83** (50): 24–7.

O'Donohue, J. (1997) *Anam Cara: Spiritual Wisdom from the Celtic World*. Bantam Press, London.

Oleson, V. & Whittaker, E. W. (1970) *The Silent Dialogue: A Study of the Social Psychology of Professional Socialization*. Jossey-Bass, San Francisco.

Packard, J. S. & Ferrara, M. (1987) In search of a moral foundation of nursing. *Advances in Nursing Science* **10** (4): 60–71.

Parker, R. (1990) Nurses' stories: the search for a relational ethic of care. *Advances in Nursing Science* **13** (1): 31–40.

Parse, R.R. (1987) Parse's Man-Living-Health theory of nursing. In *Nursing Science: Major Paradigms, Theories, and Critiques* (Parse, R. R., ed.). W. B. Saunders, Philadelphia.

Paterson, J. G. & Zderad, L. T. (1988) *Humanistic Nursing*. National League for Nursing, New York.

Pearson, A. (1983) *The Clinical Nursing Unit*. Heinemann Medical Books, London.

Pennebaker, J. W. (1989) Confession, inhibition, and disease. *Advances in Experimental Social Psychology* **22**: 211–44.

Pennebaker, J. W. & Susman, J. R. (1988) Disclosure of traumas and psychosomatic processes. *Social Science and Medicine* **26**: 327–32.

Pennebaker, J. W., Hughes, C. & O'Heeron, R. C. (1987) The psychophysiology of confession: linking inhibitory and psychosomatic processes. *Journal of Personality and Social Psychology* **52**: 781–93.

Pike, A. W. (1991) Moral outrage and moral discourse in nurse–physician collaboration. *Journal of Professional Nursing* **7** (6): 351–63.

Powell, J. (1989) The reflective practitioner in nursing. *Journal of Advanced Nursing* **14**: 824–32.

Prigogine, I. (1980) *From Being to Becoming*. W. H. Freeman, San Francisco.

Ramos, M. C. (1992) The nurse–patient relationship: themes and variations. *Journal of Advanced Nursing* **17**: 496–506.

Rawnsley, M. (1990) Of human bonding: the context of nursing as caring. *Advances in Nursing Science* **13**: 41–8.

Ray, M. A. (1989) The theory of bureaucratic caring for nursing practice in the organizational culture. *Nursing Administrative Quarterly* **13** (2): 31–42.

Reiman, D. J. (1986) Noncaring and caring in the clinical setting: patients' descriptions. *Topics in Clinical Nursing* **8** (2): 30–6.

Reisseter, K. & Thomas, B. (1986) Nursing care of the dying: its relationship to selected nurse characteristics. *International Journal of Nursing Studies* **23**: 39–50.

Reverby, S. (1987) A caring dilemma: womanhood and nursing in historical perspective. *Nursing Research* **36** (1): 5–11.

Rinpoche, S. (1992) *The Tibetan Book of Living and Dying*. Rider, London.

Roach, S. (1992) *The Human Act of Caring*. Canadian Hospital Association Press, Ottawa.

Robinson, C. & Thorne, S. (1984) Strengthening family interference. *Journal of Advanced Nursing* **9**: 597–602.

Rogers, C. R. (1969) *Freedom to Learn: A View of What Education Might Be*. Merrill, Columbus, OH.

Rogers, M. (1986) Science of unitary human beings. In *Explorations of Martha Rogers' Science of Unitary Human Beings* (Malinski, V., ed.) Appleton-Century-Crofts, Norwalk, CT.

Roper, N. Logan, W. & Tierney, A. J. (1980) *The Elements of Nursing*. Churchill Livingstone, Edinburgh.

Sacks, O. (1976) *Awakenings*. Pelican Books, London.

Sayre-Adams, J. and Wright, S. (1995) *The Theory and Practice of Therapeutic Touch*. Churchill Livingstone, Edinburgh.

Schön, D. A. (1983) *The Reflective Practitioner*. Avebury Press, Aldershot.

Schön, D. A. (1987) *Educating the Reflective Practioner*. Jossey-Bass, San Francisco.

Seedhouse, D. (1988) *Ethics: The Heart of Health Care*. Wiley, Chichester.

Smyth, J. (1987) *A Rationale for Teachers' Critical Pedagogy*. Deakin University Press, Geelong.

Smyth, J. M. & Pennebaker, J. W. (1999) Sharing one's story: translating emotional experiences into words as a coping tool. In *Coping: The Psychology of What Works* (Snyder, C. R., ed.) Oxford University Press, New York.

Smyth, J. M., Stone, A. A., Hurewitz, A. & Kaell, A. (1999) Effects of writing about stressful experiences on symptom reduction in patients with asthma or rheumatoid arthritis. *Journal of the American Medical Association* **281** (14): 1304–9.

Street, A. F. (1992) *Inside Nursing: A Critical Ethnography of Clinical Nursing*. State University of New York Press, New York.

Stewart, I. & Joines, V. (1987) *TA Today: A New Introduction to Transactional Analysis*. Lifespace Publishing, Nottingham and Chapel Hill.

Sutherland, L. (1994) Caring as mutual empowerment: working with the BNDU Model at Burford. In *The Burford NDU Model: Caring in Practice* (Johns, C., ed.), pp. 61–76. Blackwell Science, Oxford.

Taylor, B. J. (1992) From helper to human: a reconceptualization of the nurse as person. *Journal of Advanced Nursing Practice* **17**: 1042–9.

Thomas, K. & Kilmann, R. (1974) *Thomas Kilmann Conflict Mode Instrument*. Xicom, Tuxedo.

Thorne, S. & Robinson, C. (1988) Reciprocal trust in health care relationships. *Journal of Advanced Nursing* **13**: 782–9.

Tversky, A. & Kahneman, D. (1973) Availability: an heuristic for judging frequency and probability. *Cognitive Psychology* **3**: 207–32.

Tversky, A. & Khaneman, D. (1974) Judgement under uncertainty: heuristics and biases. *Science* **185**: 1124–31.

United Kingdom Central Council for Nursing, Midwifery and Health Visiting (1992) *Code of Professional Conduct*, 3rd edn. UKCC, London.

Vachon, M. (1987) Battle fatigue in hospice/palliative care. In *A Safer Death* Gilmore, A. & Gilmore, S., eds). Plenum Publishing, New York.

Van Hooft, S. (1987) Caring and professional commitment. *Australian Journal of Advanced Nursing* **4** (4): 29–38.

Van Manen, M. (1977) Linking ways of knowing with ways of being practical. *Curriculum Inquiry* **6** (3): 205–28.

Van Manen, M. (1990) *Researching Lived Experience*. State University of New York Press, New York.

Visinstainer, M. A. (1986) The nature of knowledge and theory in nursing. *Image: The Journal of Nursing Scholarship* **18**: 32–8.

Watson, J. (1988) *Nursing: Human Science and Human Care. A Theory of Nursing*. National League for Nursing, New York.

Watson, J. (1990) The moral failure of the patriarchy. *Nursing Outlook* **38** (2): 62–6.

Webster, D. (1985) Medical students' views of the nurse. *Nursing Research* 34 (5): 313–17.

Weinsheimer, J. C. (1985) *Gadamer's Hermeneutics: A Reading of 'Truth and Method'*. Yale University Press, New Haven.

White, A. K. (1993) The nursing process: a constraint on expert practice. *Journal of Nursing Management* 1 245–52.

White, J. (1995) Patterns of knowing: review, critique, and update. *Advances in Nursing Science* 17 (4) 73–86.

Wilkinson, J. M. (1988) Moral distress in nursing practice: experience and effect. *Nursing Forum* 23 (1): 16–29.

Wolf, Z. R. (1986) Nurses' work: the sacred and the profane. *Holistic Nursing Practice* 1 (1): 29–35.

Yarling, R. R. & McElmurray, B. J. (1986) The moral foundation of nursing. *Advances in Nursing Science* 3 (2): 63–73.

Young, A. M. (1976) *The Reflexive Universe: Evolution of Consciousness*. Robert Briggs, San Francisco.

Index